W9-DBI-227

Nursing-Sensitive Innovations in Patient Care

Editor

CECILIA ANNE KENNEDY PAGE

NURSING CLINICS OF NORTH AMERICA

www.nursing.theclinics.com

Consulting Editor
STEPHEN D. KRAU

March 2014 • Volume 49 • Number 1

ELSEVIER

1600 John F. Kennedy Boulevard • Suite 1800 • Philadelphia, Pennsylvania, 19103-2899

http://www.theclinics.com

NURSING CLINICS OF NORTH AMERICA Volume 49, Number 1
March 2014 ISSN 0029-6465, ISBN-13: 978-0-323-28714-2

Editor: Kerry Holland
Developmental Editor: Casey Jackson

Nursing Clinics of North America (ISSN 0029-6465) is published quarterly by Elsevier Inc., 360 Park Avenue South, New York, NY 10010-1710. Months of issue are March, June, September, and December. Periodicals postage paid at New York, NY and additional mailing offices. Subscription price per year is, $150.00 (US individuals), $400.00 (US institutions), $275.00 (international individuals), $488.00 (international institutions), $220.00 (Canadian individuals), $488.00 (Canadian institutions), $85.00 (US students), and $135.00 (international students). To receive student/resident rate, orders must be accompanied by name of affiliated institution, date of term, and the signature of program/residency coordinator on institution letterhead. Orders will be billed at individual rate until proof of status is received. Foreign air speed delivery is included in all *Clinics* subscription prices. All prices are subject to change without notice. **POSTMASTER:** Send address changes to *Nursing Clinics*, Elsevier Health Sciences Division, Subscription Customer Service, 3251 Riverport Lane, Maryland Heights, MO 63043. **Customer Service: Telephone: 1-800-654-2452** (U.S. and Canada); **1-314-447-8871 (outside U.S. and Canada). Fax: 1-314-447-8029. E-mail: journalscustomerservice-usa@elsevier.com** (for print support) and **journalsonlinesupport-usa@elsevier.com** (for online support).

Nursing Clinics of North America is covered in *EMBASE/Excerpta Medica, MEDLINE/PubMed (Index Medicus), Social Sciences Citation Index, Current Contents, ASCA, Cumulative Index to Nursing, RNdex Top 100,* and Allied Health Literature and International Nursing Index (INI).

Printed in the United States of America.

Contributors

CONSULTING EDITOR

STEPHEN D. KRAU, PhD, RN, CNE
Associate Professor, Vanderbilt University Medical Center, School of Nursing, Nashville, Tennessee

EDITOR

CECILIA ANNE KENNEDY PAGE, DNP, RN-BC, CPHIMS, PMP, FACHE
Executive Director, Informatics and Interim CIO, University of Kentucky HealthCare, Lexington, Kentucky

AUTHORS

JANE J. ABANES, DNP, RN, PMHCNS, PMHNP
Psychiatric Mental Health Nurse Practitioner and Head, Substance Abuse Rehabilitation Program, Department of Mental Health, Naval Health Clinic Hawaii, Joint Base Pearl Harbor-Hickam, Hawaii

SUSIE ADAMS, PhD, RN, PMHNP, FAANP
Professor and Director, Psychiatric Mental Health Nurse Practitioner Program, Vanderbilt University School of Nursing, Nashville, Tennessee

PENNE ALLISON, RN, BSN, MSOM, NE-BC
Director of Emergency Services, University of Kentucky HealthCare, Lexington, Kentucky

JILL BLAKE, RN, MSN
Nursing Professional Development, University of Kentucky Chandler Medical Center, Lexington, Kentucky

LACEY BUCKLER, DNP, RN, ACNP-BC, NE-BC
University of Kentucky, Lexington, Kentucky

LINDA CLEMENTS, APRN, CCNS
Cardiovascular Clinical Nurse Specialist, Nursing Professional Practice, University of Kentucky Chandler Medical Center, Lexington, Kentucky

OLGA DAYTS, DNP, RN, ACNP-BC, CCRN
Vanderbilt University Medical Center, Nashville, Tennessee

NANCYE R. FEISTRITZER, DNP, RN
Associate Hospital Director, Vanderbilt University Hospital, Nashville, Tennessee

JENNIFER FORMAN, RN, BSN
Patient Care Manager, Critical Care Services, Good Samaritan Hospital, University of Kentucky HealthCare, Lexington, Kentucky

AMANDA GREEN, DNP, RN
University of Kentucky, Lexington, Kentucky

KAREN A. HANDE, DNP, ANP-BC
Instructor of Nursing, Vanderbilt University, Nashville, Tennessee

PATRICIA KUNZ HOWARD, PhD, RN, CEN, CPEN, NE-BC, FAEN, FAAN
Operations Manager, Emergency Services, University of Kentucky Chandler Medical Center, Lexington, Kentucky

THERESE JAMISON, DNP, ACNP-BC
Associate Professor, Madonna University, Livonia, Michigan

PAM O. JONES, DNP, RN, NEA-BC
Chief Nursing Officer, Vanderbilt University Hospital, Nashville, Tennessee

NANETTE LAVOIE-VAUGHAN, MSN, ANP-C, DNP
Clinical Assistant Professor, East Carolina University College of Nursing Graduate Program, Raleigh, North Carolina

GAIL A. LIS, DNP, ACNP-BC
Associate Professor, Madonna University, Livonia, Michigan

MARY MOORE, RN, BSN
Quality and Safety Department, University of Kentucky Chandler Medical Center, Lexington, Kentucky

CECILIA KENNEDY PAGE, DNP, RN-BC, CPHIMS, PMP, FACHE
Executive Director, Informatics and Interim CIO, University of Kentucky HealthCare, Lexington, Kentucky

MATTHEW PROUD, BSN, RN, CEN
Patient Care Manager, Emergency Services, University of Kentucky Chandler Medical Center, Lexington, Kentucky

ARIC SCHADLER, PhD(ABD)
Senior Business Intelligence Analyst and Statistician, University of Kentucky HealthCare, Lexington, Kentucky

THOMAS TRIBBLE
MCS Mechanical Circulatory Support Specialist, University of Kentucky Chandler Medical Center, Lexington, Kentucky

Contents

> The quest for decreased cost of care and improved outcomes has created
> the need for highly effective clinical roles and teams. This article describes
> the role of a unit-based advanced practice registered nurse (APRN) within
> a proof-of-concept implementation of a new care delivery model, the
> Vanderbilt Anticipatory Care Team. Role clarity is central to both structural
> empowerment of the APRN and team effectiveness. A modified Peace-
> Health Team Development Measure tool measured baseline role clarity
> as a component of overall team effectiveness. A role description for the
> unit-based APRN based on a comprehensive assessment of the proof-
> of-concept unit is provided.

> A gastroenterology practice lacked quality measures to evaluate the prac-
> tice's colorectal cancer prevention efforts. Colonoscopy performance data
> were gathered from a retrospective review of 90 charts using a modified
> Colorectal Cancer Prevention Data Collection Form. Practice stakeholders
> and project leader reviewed the data, identified practice deficiencies,
> conducted root cause analysis, and developed practice changes. Imple-
> menting the prioritized recommendations and routinely benchmarking
> care was warranted to ensure effective practice to improve outcomes
> for colorectal cancer prevention. Achieving higher-value care has led to
> increased efforts to improve systems for measuring care, using these
> measures for quality improvement and directly linking quality outcomes
> to reimbursement.

> Evidence exists that patients requiring neurologic ICU admission have
> concomitant immunosuppression that makes them more prone to acquir-
> ing nosocomial infections. The risk of infection is highest in the acute phase
> after stroke, which may be attributed to stroke-induced immunodepression

syndrome. Significant numbers of patients are being diagnosed inappropriately with catheter-associated urinary tract infection, for which they receive treatment that is not recommended. Protocol-based care enables providers to translate evidence into practice.

To ensure The Joint Commission and Centers of Medicare and Medicaid Services core measures were being met, University of Kentucky Health Care created a team to explore the issues and create solutions. Six nurses were placed in the role of core measure nurse, who were responsible for identification of Core Measure patients, standard work, concurrent review, and working with the informaticist team to increase core measure performance. Building strong relationships with the bedside staff was also a key step to the success of these nurses. After the pilot, the compliance perfection scores were sustained as the roles were adopted by administration and made permanent.

Pain is the number 1 reason patients seek care in an emergency department (ED). A limiting factor for effective pain management may be clinical staff attitudes about pain and pain management. Analysis of data from an investigation into pain, perceptions, and perceived conflicts of ED staff pain management revealed a need for change. Operation Pain and ED pain champions created an environment that promoted enhanced pain management resulting in measurable outcomes. Emergency nurses participating in Operation Pain placed a higher priority on pain management for their patients.

This article describes three strategies a cardiovascular-thoracic intensive care unit implemented to decrease the rate of hospital-acquired pressure ulcers in patients on extracorporeal membranous oxygenation support. These strategies include increased staff awareness of physiologic factors placing a critically ill patient on extracorporeal support at increased risk for development of pressure ulcers, development of a turning guideline and a skin care bundle, and use of coaching by a clinical nurse specialist to promote pressure ulcer prevention.

Concept mapping and simulation provide professional nurses in the academic and practice environment with an opportunity for experiential learning. This integral combination allows for learning to be congruent with the national clinical practice guidelines that support and promote nurse-sensitive indicators. Implications for practice are forthcoming as data are collected on the impact on health outcomes when using concept mapping and simulation.

Achieving the healthcare reform goals of broad electronic medical record (EMR) adoption and meaningful use will require that usability of EMR's be addressed. A usability checklist was implemented in a process improvement redesign of nursing documentation in an academic medical center to ensure optimal design of the user interface in the EMR. The outcomes of this framework were based on metrics of usability: efficiency, effectiveness and satisfaction. Implementation of a usability checklist as standard work ensures a focus on the user interface design to enhance use of the EMR by nursing in clinical care and improve patient outcomes.

Patient satisfaction is imperative in providing safe, effective, and quality patient care. Several articles have examined the effect of a secure on-line communication system in the primary care setting to improve the delivery of patient care. This article describes the use of an asynchronous Web-based messaging system in the psychiatric outpatient setting to enhance patient satisfaction among active duty military service members.

The purpose of this project was to analyze the clinical practice guidelines for management of long-term care residents with dementia and draft an adaptation for implementation. The adaptation focused on individualizing interventions derived from evidence-based research and included strategies to maximize staff buy-in and implementation. The overall goal of the guideline is to decrease psychotropic medication use, particularly antipsychotics.

NURSING CLINICS OF NORTH AMERICA

FORTHCOMING ISSUES

June 2014
Facilitating Aging in Place: Safe, Sound, and Secure
Barbara J. Holtzclaw, PhD, RN, FAAN, and Lazelle E. Benefield, PhD, RN, FAAN, *Editors*

September 2014
Evidence-Based Practice Program
Debra Mark, PhD, RN,
Marita Titler, PhD, RN, FAAN, and Renee Latimer, APRN-BC, MS, MPH, *Editors*

December 2014
Evidence-Based Reviews in Policy and Practice
Alan Pearson, AM MSc, PhD, FCN, FAAG, FRCN, FAAN, *Editor*

RECENT ISSUES

December 2013
Genomics
Stephen D. Krau, PhD, RN, CNE, *Editor*

September 2013
Nursing and Addictions
Albert Rundio Jr, *Editor*

June 2013
Pediatrics
Patricia V. Burkhart, PhD, RN, *Editor*

RELATED INTEREST

Critical Care Nursing Clinics, June 2014, 26:2
Quality
Rosemary Luquire, RN, PhD, FAAN, NEA-BC, and Bobbi Leeper, MN, *Editors*

NOW AVAILABLE FOR YOUR iPhone and iPad

Foreword

Nurse-Sensitive Outcomes: Indicators of Quality Care?

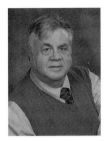

Stephen D. Krau, PhD, RN, CNE
Consulting Editor

> *Constant attention by a good nurse may be just as important as a major operation by a surgeon.*
>
> — *Dag Hammarskjold, diplomat*

Identifying the contribution nursing makes to patient care, and evaluating the quality of nursing to patient care, is considered to have begun when Florence Nightingale identified nursing's role in health care quality and began to measure outcomes. As a noted statistician, she used statistical methods to generate reports correlating patient outcomes to environmental conditions and practices. The collection of data to identify and evaluate nursing outcomes on patient care or a health care system is often referred to as "Nurse-Sensitive Outcomes," or "Nursing-Sensitive Indicators." Nursing-sensitive indicators identify configurations related to care and care processes, both of which in turn influence patient outcomes, either directly or indirectly. Nursing-sensitive indicators are specific to nursing and differ from medical indicators of care quality. As such, nursing outcome indicators are those outcomes most influenced by nursing care.[1] In spite of the lengthy history and the evolutionary strides made in measurement and research, there is still much to learn.

Nurses are essential to high-quality patient care. With the current emphasis of interdisciplinary collaboration to achieve optimal patient outcomes, the issues related to nurse-sensitive outcomes remain a dilemma. Recent literature reviews identify that evidence for nurse-sensitive outcomes is scant and somewhat nebulous due to variant measurement standards and definitions.[2] In the current health care milieu, the importance of nurse staffing and its impact on patient care and patient mortality continues to be a strong focus related to outcomes and nursing.[3,4]

The value of any health care profession is a culmination of a variety of factors that are directed at improving the management, through patient and fiscal outcomes, and

Nurs Clin N Am 49 (2014) ix–x
http://dx.doi.org/10.1016/j.cnur.2013.12.002
0029-6465/14/$ – see front matter © 2014 Published by Elsevier Inc.

nursing.theclinics.com

through funding of health services that justify the service, however measured, and the purchase of these services based on result. As a profession, nursing has had a direct effect on these outcomes. In this context, ongoing reflection about the value and contribution of nursing has been established and demonstrates that nurses contribute to promote the transformation of health systems. This mandates continual identification of nursing's contribution to the health system and, particularly, in relation to patient and health care system outcomes. There is an ongoing demand to identify and evaluate measures that allow nurses to validate responsibility for their contribution.[5]

Currently, the National Data Base of Nursing Quality Indicators (NDNDQI) is the sole national nursing data base that provides quarterly and annual reporting of structure, process, and outcome indicators to evaluate the contribution nursing makes. Currently over 1100 facilities in the United States contribute to this growing database.[1] The NDNDQI was established in 1998 by the American Nurses Association. The organization has contributed to research that is ongoing and demonstrates the distinct contribution that nurses make to the overall health care system and patient outcomes.

As we celebrate the value of interdisciplinary patient care management, it is important to consider the distinct contributions of the professions that make up this configuration. There is less information available about the efficacy of newer interdisciplinary models than there is related to nurse-sensitive indicators. This issue will illuminate some of the distinct contributions that nurses make to patient care and the health care system.

Stephen D. Krau, PhD, RN, CNE
Vanderbilt University Medical Center
School of Nursing, 461 21st Avenue South
Nashville, TN 37240, USA

E-mail address:
steve.krau@vanderbilt.edu

REFERENCES

1. Montalvo I. The National Database of Nursing Quality Indicators ® (NDNQI®). Online J Issues Nurs 2007;12(3).
2. Burston S, Chaboyer W, Gillespie B. Nurse-sensitive indicators suitable to reflect nursing care quality: a review and discussion of issues. J Clin Nurs 2013. [Epub ahead of print]. http://dx.doi.org/10.1111/jocn.12337.
3. Cho SH, Hwang JH, Kim J. Nurse staffing and patient mortality in intensive care units. Nurs Res 2008;57(5):322–30.
4. Kane RL, Shamliyan TA, Mueller C, et al. The association of registered nurse staffing levels and patient outcomes: systematic review and meta-analysis. Med Care 2007;45(12):1195–204.
5. Planas-Campmany C, Icart-Isern MT. Nursing-sensitive indicadors: an opportunity for measuring the nurse contribution. Enferm Clin 2013.

Preface

Nursing-Sensitive Innovations Influencing Outcomes

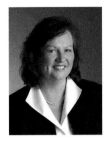

Cecilia Anne Kennedy Page, DNP, RN-BC, CPHIMS, PMP, FACHE
Editor

The changing landscape of health care today is ever challenging and calls for creativity, vision, and new models of care delivery. Emerging leaders are accepting the challenge by creating innovative strategies to transform traditional health care practices for success in the new system. This issue of *Nursing Clinics of North America* provides a view of nursing-sensitive innovations spanning various settings of care and disciplines of practice. The common thread is the innovations challenging the status quo and pushing the practice of nursing to the next frontier. Each author links the practice changes to enhanced outcomes, demonstrating the nursing contribution to the changing health care landscape.

This issue begins with a new emerging care delivery model focused on structural empowerment of the advanced practice registered nurse (APRN) and team effectiveness. These authors focused on the changing role of the APRN and its impact on patient care. Role changes are carried forth in other work, developing a core measure role for nursing. This role emphasizes the development of standardized work in meeting core measure performance, resulting in enhanced quality outcomes and data transparency for one organization. These are two examples of the emergence of new roles for nursing to influence the future of health care.

Other innovations are described in risk assessments, protocol development and implementation, and compliance to best practices in care. In each of these publications, the nurse leader challenges the current practice and emphasizes the value of using evidence-based approaches to improve practice. Carrying this one step further, one author addressed effective pain management through evaluation of staff perceptions and perceived conflicts. This analysis demonstrates that patient safety is enhanced through challenging existing clinical practices, critical thinking, and advances in care.

Nurs Clin N Am 49 (2014) xi–xii
http://dx.doi.org/10.1016/j.cnur.2013.12.001
0029-6465/14/$ – see front matter © 2014 Elsevier Inc. All rights reserved.

nursing.theclinics.com

Finally, this publication shifts to innovations in technology and the utilization of technology to optimize patient outcomes. From the approach of combining two learning strategies of concept mapping and simulation to strengthen meaningful learning to redesigning an electronic medical record to more efficiently document nursing practice, these authors present innovative opportunities to reexamine disruptive innovations and realign these technologies to enhance outcomes.

The authors in this publication are dedicated to changing health care through the advancement of nursing practice. It is my pleasure to present to you Nursing-Sensitive Innovations in Patient Care. May one of these articles change your perspective and practice as we lead the way through the health care crisis.

Cecilia Anne Kennedy Page, DNP, RN-BC, CPHIMS, PMP, FACHE
Information Technology Services
University of Kentucky HealthCare
900 South Limestone Street
Charles T. Wethington Building, Suite 317
Lexington, KY 40536-0200, USA

E-mail address:
Cecilia.page@uky.edu

A Proof-of-Concept Implementation of a Unit-Based Advanced Practice Registered Nurse (APRN) Role

Structural Empowerment, Role Clarity and Team Effectiveness

Nancye R. Feistritzer, DNP, RN*, Pam O. Jones, DNP, RN, NEA-BC

KEYWORDS

- Structural empowerment • Role clarity • Team effectiveness • Anticipatory care
- APRN role

KEY POINTS

- Role clarity is an important element of advanced practice registered nurse (APRN) structural empowerment and overall team effectiveness.
- The PEPPA framework was used to develop role specific delineation of the APRN role as a unit-based provider for the Vanderbilt Anticipatory Care Team care delivery model proof of concept.
- A modified PeaceHealth Team Development Measure was used to measure baseline team effectiveness.

Improving the US health care delivery system is a national priority. Patient care within the US health care system is often reactive and unreliable, resulting in escalating health care costs and inherent inefficiencies in the current system. As the recent Institute of Medicine (IOM) report revealed, patients are at significant risk of harm from hospital-acquired conditions and medical errors. Significant attention by the health care industry over the past decade has been focused on efficiency, quality, safety, and the implementation of evidence-based care. This has forced an evaluation and redesign of care delivery models throughout the continuum of care. Nursing leadership holds the call to action to create innovative models of care delivery to provide safe and efficient quality care.

Disclosures: The authors have no funding sources or conflict of interest to disclose.
Vanderbilt University Hospital, Hospital Administration, MCN AA-1204 21st Aveune South, Nashville, TN 37232, USA
* Corresponding author.
E-mail address: nancye.feistritzer@vanderbilt.edu

Nurs Clin N Am 49 (2014) 1–13
http://dx.doi.org/10.1016/j.cnur.2013.11.009
0029-6465/14/$ – see front matter © 2014 Elsevier Inc. All rights reserved.
nursing.theclinics.com

Despite recent efforts, health care spending remains high and accepted measures of health outcomes remain relatively poor.[1] The United States ranks the highest on health care spending per capita in a comparison of 30 industrialized countries.[1] This spending has not contributed to significant improvement in life expectancy, which ranks in the bottom quartile.[1] The United States also has the highest rate of mortality amenable to health care, which is further evidence of a failed system.[1]

Large-scale health care reform and improvement efforts are important to create a culture of improvement and innovation. The effective execution of most improvement efforts, however, occurs within clinical microsystems, such as at the nursing unit or intensive care unit level within a large hospital.[2] The Vanderbilt Anticipatory Care Team (vACT) is an improvement effort within a medical-surgical clinical microsystem that has the potential to significantly impact the organization's care delivery model.

VACT

Vanderbilt University Medical Center (VUMC) embarked on the development of a new care delivery model, vACT, to address the deficiencies inherent in the existing system of care. Nursing leadership challenged the status quo of care and created a model focused on change. The aim of the vACT project is to create improvements in patient care delivery by embedding highly effective teams, process, and informatics tools within the clinical microsystem. A conceptual model depicting vACT across the patient care continuum is included (**Fig. 1**).

The initial proof of concept of vACT is focused on the inpatient setting from June 2013 to present on an adult surgical nursing unit. The proof of concept interventions include the following:

- An advanced practice registered nurse (APRN) functioning in a unit-based provider role

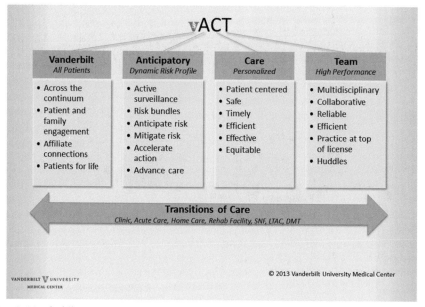

Fig. 1. Vanderbilt Anticipatory Care Team vision. (© 2013 Vanderbilt University Medical Center).

- Structured communication huddles
- Coordinated activities with intervention teams to provide targeted interventions based on patient specific need
- Role clarification and team training for increased communication, efficiency and reliability
- And the use of a dynamic risk profile (DRP) to anticipate care needs

A comprehensive discussion of the broad vACT project is outside the scope of this article. The concept of role clarity of the APRN unit-based provider, structured communication, and team effectiveness, however, are central to the vACT care delivery model and are described here. The position of the unit-based team relative to the patient is represented in **Fig. 2**.

STRUCTURAL EMPOWERMENT

A fundamental component of the vACT model is enhancement of the unit-based care team that is geographically located on the inpatient unit. The intent is for an APRN to lead this enhanced unit-based team. Although the unit-based APRN within the context of vACT is a new role for the medical center, this role has been introduced in the literature.

Cowan and colleagues[3] published a study of the effectiveness of a unit-based APRN working in collaboration with a physician-hospitalist to manage patients on a general medicine unit in an academic medical center. Acutely ill medical patients (n = 1207) were assigned to experimental and control units based on the hospital standard bed assignment routine.[3] Interventions included increased physician collaboration with the unit-based APRN and daily multidisciplinary rounds.[3] The results of the study included a decreased length of stay by 1 day and an increase in net profit

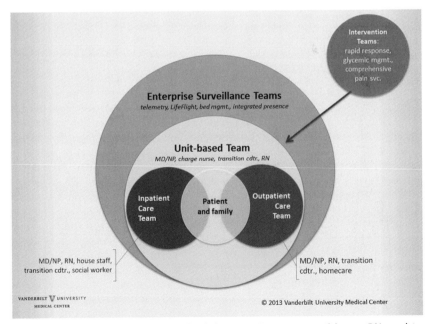

Fig. 2. vACT team structure. MD, medical doctor; NP, nurse practitioner; RN, registered nurse. (© 2013 Vanderbilt University Medical Center).

of $1591 for each patient in the experimental group.[3] There was no statistically significant difference between the 2 groups in the proportion of patients who died over the course of 4 months ($P = .31$).[3] This study provides some preliminary evidence in support of a model of care including a unit-based APRN by providing efficient care at a lower cost.

The significance of this new model of care for nursing and advanced practice nursing is clear. This model creates nursing roles that are consistent with the IOM recommendations related to nurses working at the highest level of their education and training.[4] The vACT project promotes an interprofessional team with important roles for APRNs, staff nurses, charge nurses, and nurse leaders. The opportunity for development of APRNs is particularly significant through the key roles envisioned on the unit-based team and the dynamic intervention teams. The expanded roles are in complete alignment with the IOM recommendations.[4]

Hiring a well-qualified APRN and placing that individual within the proof-of-concept unit team will not be enough to ensure success of the person, or the role. Structural empowerment, including careful role definition, is required for the implementation and sustainability of this APRN role. Role clarity is an important contributor and must be considered before implementation of a new APRN role.[5] In addition, the APRN must function as a member of a highly effective team.

The concept of structural empowerment is based on the work of Kanter,[6,7] related to the organizational characteristics and circumstances that contribute to employees being empowered. In Kanter's publications,[6,7] she described the Theory of Structural Power in Organizations, which is the seminal work for subsequent evidence. The basis for the theory is that employees derive power through formal and informal structures in the workplace. The concepts associated with structural empowerment are foundational to the design and implementation of the unit-based APRN role and provide an important conceptual framework for this project. The organizational structure, leadership structure, physician relationships, role function of the unit-based APRN, and support requirements must all be considered. Role definition is of particular importance.

DEFINITION OF THE UNIT-BASED APRN ROLE

Bryant-Lukosius and Dicenso[5] conceptualized a framework for implementation and evaluation of APRN roles (PEPPA) that is logically congruent with the principles of structural empowerment. The PEPPA framework provides a "participatory, evidence-based, patient-centered process, for APN role development, implementation, and evaluation."[5] PEPPA resulted from the authors' synthesis of frameworks introduced previously by Spitzer[8] and Dunn and Nicklin,[9] and related literature. The framework uses the principles of participatory action research (PAR), which is described as a methodology that actively involves individuals or communities in a process to design and evaluate change.[5]

The design and implementation of the unit-based APRN occurred within the implementation of the proof of concept unit for vACT, an inpatient orthopedic unit. The first 6 steps of the PEPPA framework were used by an implementation team to define the APRN role functions (**Box 1**). The implementation team included nursing leaders, physician leaders, staff nurses, representatives from nursing education, a PhD-prepared nurse who is a quality and safety expert, and a consultant in patient transition management. In addition, both authors served on this team in a facilitative role.

There was also a need to capture the perspective of a broader group of those individuals or groups who were likely to be impacted by the change, or stakeholders.[5]

> **Box 1**
> **PEPPA framework steps**
>
> Step 1 – Define patient population and describe model of care
>
> Step 2 – Identify stakeholders and recruit participants
>
> Step 3 – Determine need for a new model of care
>
> Step 4 – Identify priority problems and goals
>
> Step 5 – Define the new model of care and APRN role
>
> Step 6 – Plan implementation strategies
>
> Step 7 – Initiate APRN role implementation plan
>
> Step 8 – Evaluate APRN role and new model of care
>
> Step 9 – Long-term monitoring of the APN role and model of care
>
> *Adapted from* Bryant-Lukosius D, Dicenso A. A framework for the introduction and evaluation of advanced practice nursing roles. J Adv Nurs 2004;48(5):530–40; with permission.

Stakeholders in this project included a variety of members of the interprofessional team who were not members of the participant group. Interactive meetings were conducted with key stakeholders, such as the unit medical director and other orthopedic physicians. Collaboration with key stakeholders enabled iterative improvement and further innovation as the model was enhanced.

Extensive qualitative data were obtained through stakeholder and participant observations and discussions. The unit-specific implementation team, consistent with the principles of PAR embedded in the PEPPA framework, reviewed and analyzed these data through participative team discussions. Quantitative data that were reviewed by the implementation team included unit adverse events, rapid response team calls, patient satisfaction, and nursing-sensitive measures. The purpose of this analysis was to determine gaps in the current care processes and team functions that could be improved by the unit-based APRN role.

The resultant role description for the unit-based APRN represents a synthesis of the qualitative and quantitative information obtained through the application of the PEPPA framework (**Box 2**). A workflow map of a typical day for the APRN is also included (**Fig. 3**). The workflow and role functions were developed to meet identified opportunities for improvement in care delivery and team communication. The focus on highly effective communication and the use of informatics tools is intended to anticipate patient problems and prevent them before they occur. As of November 2013 during the proof of concept implementation, the unit-based APRN is fully functional. Evaluation of the impact on patient outcomes is pending.

TEAM EFFECTIVENESS

The success of the vACT project is not just dependent on one rule, but rather requires a highly effective team. A team is 2 or more people, who interact dynamically, interdependently, and adaptively toward a common and valued goal; have specific roles or functions; and have a time-limited membership.[10] Health care team attributes are an important consideration when seeking optimal effectiveness. The composition of the team, level of empowerment, accountability for outcomes, and power gradient all affect the quality of team interactions.[11] In the end, teams are composed of

---

Box 2
Unit-based APRN role description

Primary Role Functions

The unit-based APRN will function within the scope of practice as defined by state licensure and organizational rules and regulations. Competency validation will be conducted per routine Focused Professional Practice Evaluation (FPPE) and Ongoing Professional Practice Evaluation (OPPE) processes.

The APRN will function as a member of the interprofessional unit-based team. The team will be trained in structured communication processes as part of the vACT proof of concept implementation. The unit-based APRN will use specific strategies to coordinate care including huddles, briefings, debriefs and Subject Background Analysis Recommendation (SBAR) communication tools. A priority is creating a culture of safety and continuous improvement in collaboration with local management, medical staff, and hospital administration.

The APRN will participate in daily team transition huddles as part of enhanced communication and coordination of discharge planning. The dynamic risk profile will be used as a communication tool during these huddles.

Other priority activities are defined by the identified needs of the patients, families, and stakeholders. The following are areas of focus based on these identified needs:

- Diagnosis and treatment as appropriate per scope of APRN license.
- Face-to-face rounding on all patients to improve communication and facilitate resolution of issues. This rounding should be done with a bedside nurse whenever possible. Initial priority items should be pain control, understanding of the plan of care, resolution of patient/family questions or concerns, and readiness for discharge.
- Use of the dynamic risk profile as an informatics tool to promote situational awareness of patients on the unit and anticipate care.
- Ensure completion of the "first possible discharge date" data field to promote proactive planning for discharge on the part of the team.
- Participate in daily interprofessional transition huddles.
- Participate in structure handovers with the night shift charge nurse at the beginning of the shift.
- Conduct or participate in debriefs after any adverse events or significant unanticipated problems.
- Focus on completion of medication reconciliation on patients on the unit as appropriate.
- Coordinate with consulting services on the unit and ensure enhanced communication and appropriate orders are written in a timely manner.
- Timely completion of discharge summaries and orders for primary patients. Assist nursing staff in facilitating completion of off-service patients.
- Participate in the development and advancement of an interprofessional falls-prevention with special attention to the implications of medications on falls risk.
- Focus on documentation of pressure ulcers present on admission for new admissions (POA).

Conduct debrief of any readmissions to the unit.

---

individuals. Each team member must feel a personal sense of empowerment, engagement, and accountability to the rest of the team and to patients for the outcomes associated with their efforts. For example, "a strategy that entrusts and empowers nurses to manage their own capacity for patient care is a 'win' for both nurses and patients".[12]

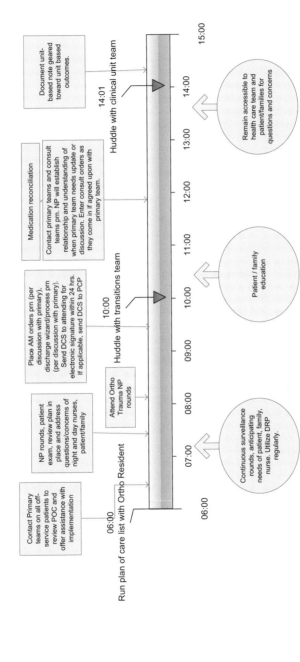

Fig. 3. Unit-based NP sample workday.

To work effectively together, team members must possess "specific knowledge, skills, and attitudes (KSAs) such as skill in monitoring each other's performance, knowledge of their own and teammates' task responsibilities, and a positive disposition toward working in a team."[13] This was of particular importance in the development of the new unit-based APRN role. There are 3 major categories of KSAs required by members of the vACT proof of concept team:

- Establishment of the organization and administration of the team is required to define the team leadership, develop clear role delineation, define behavioral markers of teamwork skills, and provide education, simulation, and transfer of knowledge systems.
- Clinical competence and decision-making authority must be present with recognition of the need for emotional intelligence, adaptive coordination of nonroutine events, and recognition of human performance limitations.
- Personal empowerment grounded in interpersonal skills, collaboration, and professional interactions are essential to effective health care teams. Sentinel event analysis often reveals that someone on the team recognized that something was going wrong. That individual was often too intimidated to speak up and alert the team. The empowerment to "See it and Say it" is an essential component to effective team communication. The team should use interactive communication protocols to enable individual members to both say what they think and to provide cues for the members of the team to stop and listen.

COMPONENTS OF TEAM DEVELOPMENT

Team effectiveness is essential to the provision of health care in the inpatient acute care setting. Inpatient medical-surgical units are increasingly complex as the acuity of hospitalized patients increases.[14] Historically, physicians, nurses, and other health care professionals have functioned as discrete entities on such units. Subsequent to its assessment of and recommendations for the American health system in 1999 and 2001, the IOM recommended that interdisciplinary team training programs be established, based on sound principles of team management, to improve coordination and communication among health care staff.[13,15–17]

The PeaceHealth System is a faith-based health system in the northwest United States. Leaders from PeaceHealth focused on team development to enable implementation of improvement initiatives undertaken by the system. The Team Development Measure (TDM) (**Box 3**) was developed to measure readiness for improvement activities in the system.[18] Team development is the degree to which a team possesses the components needed for highly effective teamwork and how firmly these components are in place. The TDM measures 4 components of team development: cohesiveness, communication, role clarity, and goals and means clarity.

Cohesiveness

The initial component as a team develops is cohesiveness (attraction of the members to the team). Cohesiveness is the social glue that binds the team members together as a unit. Without cohesiveness, it is extremely difficult for a team to attain the other components of a developed team.

Communication

The next component of team development to be put in place is communication. Communication involves the full range of topics, including decision-making and problem solving. Communication can be a difficult process and thus rests on the

Box 3
PeaceHealth Team development measure

1. Team members say what they really mean.

2. Team members say what they really think.

3. Team members talk about other team members behind their back.

4. All team members participate in making decisions about the work of the team.

5. All team members feel free to share their ideas with the team.

6. All team members feel free to express their feelings with the team.

7. The team practices tolerance flexibility and appreciation of the unique differences between team members.

8. The team handles conflicts in a calm, caring, and healing manner.

9. Regardless of the topic, communication between the people on this team is direct, truthful, respectful, and positive.

10. The team openly discusses decisions that affect the work of the team before they are made.

11. In this team, members support, nurture, and care for each other.

12. The team has agreed on clear criteria for evaluating the outcomes of the team's effort.

13. As a team, we come up with creative solutions to problems.

14. In the team, there is more of a WE feeling than an ME feeling.

15. There is confusion about what the work is that the team should be doing.

16. There is confusion about how to accomplish the work of the team.

17. Roles and responsibilities of individual team members are clearly understood by all members of the team.

18. All team members place the accomplishments of the team ahead of their own individual accomplishments.

19. The goals of the team are clearly understood by all team members.

20. All team members define the goals of the team as more important than their own personal goals.

21. I am happy with the outcomes of the team's work so far.

22. I enjoy being in the company of the other members of the team.

23. This team is a personally meaningful experience for me.

24. I have a clear understanding of what other team members expect of me as a team member.

25. The work I do on this team is valued by the other team members.

26. I am allowed to use my unique personal skills and abilities for the benefit of the team.

27. Some members of this team resist being led.

28. Information that is important for the team to have is openly shared by and with all team members.

29. All individuals on this team feel free to suggest ways to improve how the team functions.

30. When team problems arise, the team openly explores options to solve them.

31. On this team, the person who takes the lead differs depending on who is best suited for the task.

Courtesy of PeaceHealth, Vancouver, WA; with permission. Available at: http://www.peacehealth.org/about-peacehealth/medical-professionals/eugene-springfield-cottage-grove/team-measure/Pages/measure.aspx. Accessed October 1, 2013.

team having a certain level of cohesiveness for that communication to occur. Communication is, of course, central, as further team development and effective functioning simply cannot occur without team communication.

Role Clarity

The next component to become part of the team is clear role definitions and expectations. Here team members take on the role of "Team Member" as a primary role. The role of team member supersedes individual roles that team members bring with them into the team. Although the professional roles brought to the team are what give the team its potential strength, these professional roles must be defined by team members as equal in importance as the role of team member if the team is to fully develop. Additionally, team members know who is doing what and what the other team members expect of them.

Goals and Means Clarity

The final component of team development to become a team attribute is clearly defined team goals and the means to reach these goals.[18]

STAGES OF TEAM DEVELOPMENT

As a team moves from a collection of individuals to a fully developed team, the 4 general components of team development become part of the team. The transition to a fully developed team involves the solidification of the 4 components. In the process of becoming fully developed, these components become present in the team, but are initially not firmly in place. When a team has developed to the point that components are firmly in place, the team is becoming resilient. Disruptive events, from either within or outside of the team, are taken in stride as the team continues to move forward in its work.

The 4 components and 2 levels of solidification form 8 stages of team development. Thus, the voice of the team is captured. In addition, these stages, and the scores associated with each, are merely approximations and not precise points on the scale where movement to a different stage occurs. Movement from one stage to the next is more of a flow in the development of a team than it is a distinct step up the ladder of team development. Within each stage, the more the team score is toward the higher score in the range, the more of those components that are present.

DATA COLLECTION

To measure baseline performance of the patient care and unit-based team, before and after role and team training, the TDM was administered. Subsequent to Vanderbilt institutional review board approval as a quality improvement initiative and with permission to use the PeaceHealth TDM tool, members of both the patient care and unit-based team on the Proof of Concept (POC) unit received an e-mail with an imbedded link to the modified PeaceHealth TDM questionnaire.

Teams then received training from the Vanderbilt Department for Professional Development and the Center for Clinical Improvement on the vACT model, roles, and processes using the Agency for Healthcare Quality and Research TeamSTEPPS methodology.[19] The training occurred through a series of 2-hour sessions and was well received by participants based on feedback at the time of training. Computers were available at the training site to enable any attendees who had not yet completed the TDM survey to do so before the training.

DATA COLLECTION TOOL

The original PeaceHealth TDM Tool is a 31-item self-report survey with a 4-point Likert scale created. The original survey tool was modified for this POC to add a fifth response of undecided as follows:

1. Strongly disagree
2. Disagree
3. Undecided
4. Agree
5. Strongly agree

The addition of an undecided response ensured that participants were not forced to answer into either end of the scale. Because an undecided response was still not an agreement about that survey item, the undecided response was scored as a 2. The original TDM score table was then used to develop a team development score.

Scores on the TDM measure are intervals (1 point is the same size anywhere on the scale) and thus the measure literally constitutes a yardstick to measure team development. Scores range from 0 to 100, where 0 = no team development and 100 = full team development. Team development is thus how far the team is up the yardstick between no team development and full team development.[18]

Before any education, an email with a link to the TDM survey was sent to 63 unit staff, case managers, and social workers, as well as 27 service-based providers, including attending surgeons, residents, fellows, and APRNs on the surgical service. Participants completed 43 surveys for a response rate of 47.8%. A role-specific breakdown revealed that most respondents were staff nurses, which is not surprising given that they represent the largest number of members of the team. Further role-specific delineation included attending surgeon (3, 7.0%), resident (2, 4.7%), staff nurse (27, 62.8%), nurse practitioner (1, 2.3%), care partner (3, 7.0%), case manager (0, 0%), social worker (0, 0%), and other member of the care team (7, 16.3%). The lower response rates of non-nurse members of the team highlights the opportunity to further engage attending surgeons, housestaff, case managers, social workers, service-based nurse practitioners, and other members of the team.

TEAM DEVELOPMENT COMPONENTS AND SOLIDIFICATION

To understand the presence of components and the level of solidification, it is important to recognize that the definition of team for the proof of concept included all types of roles, as previously described. The individual team member perceptions produced a collective perception of the team through a Rasch analysis. A central feature of Rasch analysis is that it captures how respondents to the survey see the world. Thus, the voice of the team was captured. The team development score was 49.33 of 100, $\sigma2 = 61.93$, $\sigma = 1.20$, $t = 41.1$, confidence interval (CI) = 95%. This score places the team in Stage 2 of team development. Only 2 of the 4 components were in place at the start of the proof of concept, cohesiveness and communication, with the 2 other components, role clarity and goals and means clarity, absent. None of the 4 components was firmly in place (**Table 1**).

The unit-based proof-of-concept team has a major opportunity to further develop into a more effective care team. The team training conducted as part of the proof of concept has provided additional skills to enable the team to establish baseline skills. Areas of future emphasis and training must include further role clarity coupled with a

Stage	Score Range	Components Present	Solidification
Table 1			
Initial stage of team development for Vanderbilt Proof of Concept Unit as measured by the PeaceHealth Team Development Measure			
Pre-team	0–36	None to building cohesiveness	None
1	37–46	Cohesiveness	In place
2	47–54	Communication	
3	55–57	Role clarity	
4	58–63	Goals & means clarity	
5	64–69	Cohesiveness	Firmly in place
6	70–77	Communication	
7	78–80	Role clarity	
8	81–86	Goals & means clarity	
Fully developed	87–100	Everything	

Courtesy of PeaceHealth, Vancouver, WA; with permission. Available at: http://www.peacehealth.org/about-peacehealth/medical-professionals/eugene-springfield-cottage-grove/team-measure/Pages/measure.aspx. Accessed October 1, 2013.

more comprehensive understanding of the goals and means the team has available. In addition, the solidification of all components of the team will be an area of emphasis and development. The focus on the unit has demonstrated organizational support that is strengthening the team's understanding of the means they have available to accomplish their goals.

SUMMARY

In 2010, Maureen Bisognano, president of Institute for Healthcare Improvement (IHI) offered 6 recommendations to improve health care quality and safety through the framework of nursing. Her recommendations were as follows:

- Focus on transformational leadership at all levels
- Redesign care to optimize nurses' professional expertise and knowledge
- All hospital personnel should work together to ensure safe and reliable care for patients in acute settings
- Systems and a culture should be built that encourage, support, and spread vitality and teamwork in all areas of nursing
- Put in place structures and processes that ensure patient-centered care
- A national learning system is needed to make all models and prototypes accessible to nurses at all levels[20]

The vACT proof of concept is under way at Vanderbilt and has the potential to redesign the delivery of inpatient care. The development and implementation of this new care-delivery model meets the challenges of Bisognano's recommendations. An APRN functioning as a key member of this interprofessional team of the future provides a tremendous opportunity for advanced practice nursing to assume a leadership role. Structural empowerment and team effectiveness are important topics for the future of advanced practice nursing. As described in the IOM publication,[4] the potential for nursing is tremendous. This care delivery model is a cornerstone for advanced practice nursing and the power to improve patient outcomes through anticipation and mitigation of risk leading to a reduction in fragmentation of care.

REFERENCES

1. Anderson GF, Squires DA. Measuring the U.S. health care system: a cross-national comparison. Issue Brief (Commonw Fund) 2010;90:1–10.
2. Nelson EC. Value by design: developing clinical microsystems to achieve organizational excellence. San Francisco (CA): Jossey-Bass; 2011.
3. Cowan MJ, Shaprio M, Harris RD, et al. The effects of a multidisciplinary hospitalist/physician and advanced practice nurse collaboration on hospital costs. J Nurs Adm 2006;48(5):530–40.
4. Institute of Medicine. The future of nursing: leading change, advancing health. Washington, DC: The National Academies Press; 2011.
5. Bryant-Lukosius D, Dicenso A. A framework for the introduction and evaluation of advanced practice nursing roles. J Adv Nurs 2004;48(5):530–40.
6. Kanter RM. Men and women of the corporation. New York: Basic Books; 1977.
7. Kanter RM. Men and women of the corporation. New York: Basic Books; 1993.
8. Spitzer W. Evidence that justifies the introduction of new health professionals. In: Spitzer W, editor. The professions and public policy. Toronto: University of Toronto Press; 1978. p. 211–36.
9. Dunn K, Nicklin W. The status of advanced nursing roles in Canadian teaching hospitals. Can J Nurs Admin 1995;111–35.
10. Leggat SG. Effective health care teams require effective team members: defining teamwork competencies. BMC Health Serv Res 2007;7:17.
11. Salas E, Dickinson TL, Converse SA. Toward an understanding of team performance and training. In: Swezey RW, Salas E, editors. Teams: their training and performance. Norwood (NJ): Ablex; 1992. p. 3–29.
12. Rutherford P, Lee B, Greiner A. Transforming care at the bedside. 2004. Available at: www.ihi.org
13. Baker DP, Day R, Salas E. Teamwork as an essential component of high-reliability organizations. Health Serv Res 2006;41(4 Pt 2):1576–98.
14. Friedman DM, Berger DL. Improving team structure and communication: a key to hospital efficiency. Arch Surg 2004;139(11):1194–8.
15. Institute of Medicine. To err is human: building a safer health system. Washington, DC: The National Academies Press; 1999.
16. Institute of Medicine. Crossing the quality chasm: a new health system for the 21st century. Washington, DC: The National Academies Press; 2001.
17. Agency for Healthcare Research and Quality. Chapter 1: medical teamwork and patient safety: the evidence-based relation. 2005. Available at: http://www.ahrq.gov/research/findings/final-reports/medteam/chapter1.html. Accessed October 1, 2013.
18. PeaceHealth. Team development measure. Available at: http://www.peacehealth.org/about-peacehealth/medical-professionals/eugene-springfield-cottage-grove/team-measure/Pages/measure.aspx. Accessed October 1, 2013.
19. Agency for Healthcare Research and Quality. Patient safety primers. Available at: http://psnet.ahrq.gov/primer.aspx?primerID=5. Accessed October 1, 2013.
20. Bisognano M. Nursing's role in transforming healthcare. Nurses are crucial to closing quality-of-care gaps. Healthc Exec 2010;25(2):84, 86–7.

Measuring Endoscopic Performance for Colorectal Cancer Prevention Quality Improvement in a Gastroenterology Practice

Karen A. Hande, DNP, ANP-BC

KEYWORDS

- Colorectal cancer prevention • Quality improvement • Endoscopic performance
- DNP

KEY POINTS

- The DNP nurse explores an aspect of quality improvement while considering how to translate, evaluate, and apply science to practice.
- Studying individual or practice performance allows clinicians to identify gaps in quality, implement changes, and measure and report improvement.
- The PDSA model, TQM theoretical framework, and evidence-based measures are useful tools to guide clinicians to measure quality of care and improve health care delivery for favorable patient outcomes.

Colorectal cancer (CRC) remains the third leading cause of cancer death for men and women.[1] There has been an overall decline in CRC incidence over the past two decades, with an accelerated drop after 1998 attributed to the use of screening CRC tests and reduced exposure to risk factors. Prospective randomized trials and observational studies have demonstrated mortality reductions associated with early detection of invasive disease and removal of adenomatous polyps.[2–5] Even greater incidence and mortality reductions could be achieved in a larger proportion of adults if CRC prevention efforts were improved.[6,7]

Several experts propose that tracking care based on quality measures leads to improved outcomes for CRC prevention (CRC-P).[8,9] A data form is a useful initial tool for acquiring information about endoscopy practices and identifying deficiencies in performance. The American Gastroenterology Association Digestive Health Outcomes Registry developed such a data form, the Colorectal Cancer Prevention Data Collection Form.[10] This tool can be used to identity CRC-P poor performance areas

Disclosure Statement: The author has nothing to disclose.
Vanderbilt University, 461 21st Avenue South, Godchaux Hall #306, Nashville, TN 37240, USA
E-mail address: karen.a.hande@vanderbilt.edu

as the impetus for analyzing possible causes and developing actions to improve these areas.

Nurses can lead a culture of quality and safety by measuring and reporting their specialty area's performance. Nurses create innovative practice changes to continuously improve practice performance and patient outcomes. Finding and implementing best health care practices, or "benchmarking," is a novel approach nurses can effectively use.[11]

A nurse conducted a gastrointestinal (GI) practice analysis and identified a lack of quality measures to evaluate the practice's efforts to prevent CRC. Thus, the providers in this practice were unable to assess their quality of care against established benchmarks in the gastroenterology community at large. This created a potential barrier to meet the practice's aim to deliver safe, effective, timely, patient-centered, efficient, and equitable care.

The purpose of this scholarly project was for the nurse to assess the practice's adherence to CRC-P benchmarking measures regarding colonoscopy performance. The nurse's assessment identified performance gaps, uncovered opportunities for improvement in CRC-P, investigated root causes of deficiencies, and considered practice changes for improvement in the overall quality and effective delivery of colorectal care provided by this practice.

BACKGROUND AND SIGNIFICANCE

The American Gastroenterology Association Expert Panel identified specific desirable outcomes and care processes for CRC screening based on scientific evidence.[12] The CRC-P measures are specifically detailed into six categories to represent national benchmarks of quality care in CRC screening and surveillance: (1) identification of CRC risk, (2) endoscopic examination interval, (3) use of anesthesia professionals, (4) procedure-related complications, (5) colonoscopy assessment (procedural adequacy), and (6) adenoma detection rate.[12]

For a practice to achieve its clinical aims, it must base patient care on clinical practice guidelines.[8] However, that is not enough to maintain excellence in care. Care must be regularly evaluated to ensure a practice meets established quality standards. Initiating the use of an evaluation tool in a practice can reveal areas of opportunity for practice change. Quality measures and evidence necessary to support change cannot be considered in a vacuum.[8] It is not sufficient to just measure quality; quality improvement (QI) programs are the impetus for practice changes. Ultimately, improved quality, satisfaction, cost, and safety of care provide superior outcomes (**Fig. 1**).[13]

SYNTHESIS OF EVIDENCE RELATED TO PROBLEM
QI in Health Care

The Institute of Medicine (IOM) has identified specific nation-wide problems in terms of medical errors, wide discrepancy in outcomes, and safety.[13] Wider awareness of

Quality	Satisfaction
Superior	
Outcomes	
Safety	Cost

Fig. 1. Improved quality, satisfaction, cost, and safety of care provide superior outcomes. (*Adapted from* Institute of Medicine. Crossing the quality chasm: a new health care system for the 21st century. Washington, DC: National Academy Press; 2001; with permission.)

these failings has led to a new interest in QI. Borrowing from lessons learned in the manufacturing industry, health care has adopted concepts from total quality management (TQM) to address its problems with errors, outcomes, and safety.[14]

QI efforts have also impacted GI endoscopy. Recognizing the wide disparity in endoscopic skill and patient outcomes, various GI societies and experts collaborated to create quality indicators for endoscopic procedures initially by the US Multi-Society Task Force (USMSTF) for CRC and later, the American Society of Gastrointestinal Endoscopy and the American College of Gastroenterology Taskforce on Quality in Endoscopy (TQE).[15,16]

Appraisal of Evidence for Quality Indicators for Colonoscopy

Colonoscopy is the most effective and accepted method for CRC screening for patients aged 50 years and older.[17] However, colonoscopy still falls short of the ideal of 100% effectiveness in CRC-P. In a large case-control study, colonoscopy was associated with 50% reduction in CRC development and 60% reduction in CRC deaths.[18] Multiple factors seem to contribute to the limitations of colonoscopy effectiveness, including adequate visualization of the entire colon, diligence in examining the mucosa, and patient acceptance of the procedure.[16] Several studies have highlighted a worrisome discrepancy in colonoscopy quality, which suggests a wide variation in CRC-P efforts among endoscopists.[19–21]

To address the variation in quality, the USMSTF proposed expert consensus quality measures to define optimal endoscopic performance.[15] The TQE published data grading the level of evidence supporting each one of the quality indicators using the grading system previously published by Guyatt and colleagues.[16,22] There are 11 colonoscopy quality indicators identified in the article, but not all are pertinent to CRC-P.[16] For the purpose of this project, only the indicators pertaining to CRC-P are discussed (with the level of grading): appropriate indication (1C+), use of recommended postpolypectomy and postcancer resection surveillance intervals (1A), documentation in the procedure note of the quality of the preparation (2C), cecal intubation rates (1C), detection of adenomas in asymptomatic individuals (1C), and colonoscope withdrawal time (2C).[16]

The USMSTF recommends that every endoscopist embrace the QI process for colonoscopy practice.[15] The comprehensive list of quality indicators developed by the task force is an attempt to guide the QI process for practices. It is recognized, however, that each indicator is not applicable to every setting.[16] Each practice needs to select the most appropriate quality indicators for their individual QI process. Moreover, the proposed measures are recognized to be imperfect; however, they are useful early initiatives to help distinguish high-quality endoscopy from inappropriate and poorly performed procedures.[16] This can improve patient care, provide comparative information for consumers, and prepare for inevitable reporting requirements by Medicare.[23]

Initial CRC risk assessment

Screening colonoscopy, like any other medical procedure, requires documentation of proper indication before the procedure.[16] According to the US Preventative Task Force,[24] assessment of a patient's risk for CRC is an important component of the procedure indication. Patients age 50 and older are deemed at average risk for CRC if they have no family history of CRC and no personal history of colorectal polyps and/or CRC. Factors indicating an increased risk for CRC include a personal history of adenomatous polyps or a significant family history of CRC.[25,26] In the average-risk population, colonoscopic screening is recommended in all current guidelines at

10-year intervals.[24,26,27] In higher-risk patients, earlier and more frequent screening is advised.[24] For the purposes of this project, the project leader focused exclusively on average-risk patients.

Use of recommended postpolypectomy and postcancer surveillance interval

A personal history of adenomatous polyps is an independent risk factor for CRC. Therefore, on completion of an initial screening colonoscopy, it is incumbent on the endoscopist to document the presence or absence of colorectal polyps and outline a plan for future colorectal surveillance.[28] Failure to do so could lead to inappropriate patient management. For example, if a patient with a normal screening colonoscopy were to go undergo a repeat examination in 3 years, this would be an inappropriate use of resources and potentially put a patient at unnecessary procedural risk.[29] In a cohort of average-risk persons who underwent an initial colonoscopy with no polyps detected, a repeat colonoscopy 5 years later was not beneficial to prevent CRC.[29] Two studies of initial flexible sigmoidoscopy with normal findings showed that the protective effect of endoscopy was present for intervals of 10 years.[5,30]

Conversely, an inappropriately long interval to the next recommended colonoscopy (or failure to recommend a follow-up colonoscopy) could put the patient at increased risk for CRC. If a patient undergoing screening colonoscopy were to have multiple adenomatous polyps, he or she would then be considered at increased risk for future polyps.[31] To wait more than 5 years to recommend a patient to undergo a surveillance colonoscopy is inappropriately long and subjects the patient to increased risk for future colon cancer.[31]

Cecal intubation rates

A substantial fraction of colon polyps and colon cancer occur in the cecum and the proximal colon.[32] Therefore, it is imperative to visualize the entire colon during screening colonoscopy. In fact, one of the leading causes of missed colon cancer during a colonoscopy is failure of the endoscopist to reach the cecum.[31] Effective endoscopists should be able to visualize the cecum in greater than or equal to 95% of screening colonoscopies in a healthy adult.[33,34] Not only should the cecum be visualized, but clear photo documentation of the appendiceal orifice and ileocecal valve should be attained as evidence.[15,22]

Quality of bowel preparation

The TQE states that careful mucosal inspection is essential to effective CRC-P and reduction of cancer mortality.[16] Poor bowel preparation is a major impediment to the endoscopist's ability to find precancerous lesions.[35,36] Polyps 5 mm or larger are deemed clinically relevant.[15] If a bowel preparation fails to permit detection of polyps of this size, then the preparation must be considered inadequate.[15]

The TQE states that an endoscopist should describe the bowel preparation quality for every performed screening colonoscopy.[16] Terms such as "excellent" or "good" imply an adequate quality of preparation, whereas "fair" or "poor" indicate substandard quality. Although these terms do not have standard definitions, they are currently the standard descriptors for bowel preparation quality.[16] At least 90% of bowel preparations for screening colonoscopies should be "excellent" or "good." Failure to achieve quality preparations at this rate may reflect a quality-control issue and may indicate attention to the method of patient instruction or type of bowel preparation.[37]

Adenoma detection rate in screening colonoscopies

Adenomatous polyps, also known as adenomas, are premalignant precursors to CRC.[16] Thus, the principal goals of a screening colonoscopy are to detect and remove any adenomatous polyps to prevent CRC from developing.[15] Large screening colonoscopy trials have shown the prevalence of adenomas in healthy individuals to be approximately 25% among men and 15% among women.[38–40] Based on these studies, the TQE developed a specific measure for the quality of a colonoscopy. In the healthy screening population a skilled and thorough endoscopist should have an adenoma detection rate of 25% in male and 15% in female patients.[16] Adenoma detection rates less than this standard may indicate lower examination quality and may be a fundamental obstacle to prevent CRC.

Colonoscope withdrawal time

An endoscopist quantifies his or her colonoscope withdrawal time by measuring the time from which the colonoscope is retracted from the cecum to the anus. Evidence supports a direct relationship between colonoscope withdrawal times and adenoma detection rates.[39,41] Withdrawal times of 6 minutes or more from the cecum to the anus have demonstrated improved polyp detection rates; withdrawal of less than 5 minutes may reduce the effectiveness of CRC-P.[39,41,42] Hence, the established quality standard is based on the cited evidence that the mean withdrawal time should be 6 minutes or greater to prevent and screen for CRC.[16]

In conclusion, several studies support the recommendations of both the USMSTF and TQE.[15,16] Although the strengths of these studies are good, it should be noted that most are observational studies, not prospective or randomized trials (except for the polyp surveillance metric).

APPLICATION OF A THEORETICAL FRAMEWORK FOR PROJECT

Total Quality Management (TQM), also known as Continuous Quality Improvement (CQI), is a management philosophy and method with its origins in research. The philosophic basis of TQM assumes that problems in producing a quality product arise from poor job design, failure of leadership, or an unclear purpose.[14] TQM centers on an organization's QI efforts to improve service or products for patients and/or customers; the satisfaction of all people (customers, patients, employees, leaders) determines quality.[43] The underlying principle of TQM is people are basically good and work hard, but the system in which they work may fail them, resulting in required QI.[44]

At the root of TQM lays the use of team structure and the understanding of team dynamics. TQM entails the redesign of care processes by encouraging cycles of change and stability.[45] It is an ongoing process that requires teams of participants (stakeholders, leaders, customers, employees, management) to critically assess processes, problem solve, and implement solutions.[45] One such method used for the TQM process is the Plan-Do-Study-Act cycle (PDSA).[46]

METHODOLOGY

The PDSA[46] process was the framework for the project's design (**Fig. 2**).

Plan

A proposal was submitted to Vanderbilt University Institutional Review Board and a letter of approval was obtained. The project leader met with the three gastroenterologists to establish their investment in the project. The need for an evaluation of colonoscopy performance to prevent CRC, the modified CRC-P clinical data form, and the TQE quality metrics was described by the project leader. Finally, the project leader requested the stakeholders' agreement to meet and collectively review the data

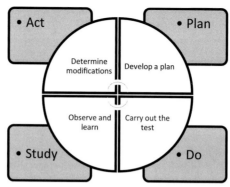

Fig. 2. Project design: plan-do-study-act framework. (*Adapted from* Langley GL, Nolan KM, Nolan TW, et al. (2009) The improvement guide: a practical approach to enhancing organizational performance (2nd edition). San Francisco: Jossey Bass; 2009.)

analysis of the practice's colonoscopy performance, identify performance gaps and root causes, and develop practice changes to implement for QI.

Do

The project leader modified the Colorectal Cancer Prevention Data Collection Form[16] for the purpose of this project. The modified collection tool included the medical record number, date of colonoscopy, endoscopist's identifier (assigned number one, two, or three), age, gender, and evidence-based TQE metrics (**Fig. 3**).

The project leader conducted a retrospective chart review of 90 colonoscopy reports. She randomly selected 30 reports per provider in the practice's electronic medical record. Each of the reports had to meet specific inclusion criteria (**Box 1**). The data were collected on the modified data collection tool and then recorded in an Excel spreadsheet.

Modified CRC-P Data Collection Form

Endoscopist Number: 1 2 3   MRN: Date of procedure:

Sex: Male   Female   Age:

Initial CRC Risk Assessment: Documented   Not Documented

Preparation Adequacy: Excellent   Good   Fair   Poor

Polyps Present or Absent: Documented   Not Documented

Recommended post-polypectomy or post-cancer surveillance time: Documented

                                                                Not Documented

Cecum Intubated: Yes   No

Adenoma detected?   Yes   No   Number detected?

Colonoscope withdrawal time from cecum: minutes   or   Not Documented

Fig. 3. Modified CRC-P data collection form.

> **Box 1**
> **Inclusion criteria**
>
> - 50 years or older
> - No prior CRC
> - Indication for the procedure a screening colonoscopy
> - Procedure performed during October 1, 2012 to December 31, 2012

Study

Descriptive statistics were used for the project leader to analyze colonoscopy performance. The percentage for each metric was calculated for endoscopist one, two, and three, and the practice as a whole. The data were then compared with the following established 2006 TQE standards and graded as "met standard" or "substandard":

- Initial CRC risk assessment must be documented for the procedure; absence of documentation is substandard performance.
- The recommended postpolypectomy and postcancer surveillance time and the presence or absence of colorectal polyps must be stated. The failure to do so is considered substandard performance.
- Cecal intubation rates should be greater than or equal to 95% of screening colonoscopies in a healthy adult; less than is substandard.
- Quality of bowel preparation should be graded as "excellent" or "good" in at least 90% of procedures; "fair" or "poor" preparations indicate substandard quality.
- Adenoma detection rate should be 25% in male patients and 15% in female patients; rates less than this are substandard.
- Mean colonoscopy withdrawal time should be 6 minutes or greater; 5 minutes or less is substandard.

Act

The project leader distributed the graded metric results to the stakeholders for individual review. The stakeholders and the project leader met to conduct a root cause analysis. The root cause analysis consisted of a group discussion of system problems leading to substandard performance. The group then mutually explored and developed practice changes to improve the system issues (**Fig. 4**).

RESULTS

Ninety reports for screening colonoscopies were randomly selected from the electronic medical record. All of the reports met the required inclusion criteria (see **Box 1**). The population demographics were identified (**Box 2**). The TQE metric

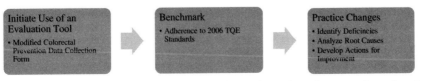

Fig. 4. Project's process of quality improvement for endoscopic performance for colorectal cancer prevention in a GI practice.

Box 2 Patient demographics		
Mean Age (Years)	**Males (N)**	**Females (N)**
57.9	43	47

standards, practice results for each metric, and the grade of each practice metric are shown in **Table 1**.

The stakeholders identified the first area of substandard performance as measurement and documentation of colonoscope withdrawal time for each procedure. The root causes for substandard performance were identified as the absence and the varying approaches for measuring and documenting colonoscope withdrawal time. One endoscopist estimated the withdrawal time. Another endoscopist stated that he simply did not calculate the time on any of his procedures. It was unanimously agreed to time every colonoscopy with a stopwatch. The endoscopy technician would be designated to start the timer when the colonoscope was being withdrawn from the cecum, stop at the withdrawal of the scope from the anus, and document the time in the procedural record.

The stakeholders identified a second area for QI to be the documentation of recommended CRC-P surveillance and the presence and absence of polyps. The root cause for this measure was that the endoscopists did not consistently include the required information as part of the assessment and plan in the colonoscopy report for each patient. They agreed to document this information routinely to meet the established standard.

The stakeholders identified a third deficiency to be the documentation of CRC risk assessments. The root cause for substandard performance was found to be the deficiency of a conducted assessment for each patient. The CRC risk assessment is not routinely done at their initial clinic visit, and is not part of the colonoscopy record. The agreed on practice initiative was to create an assessment template and incorporate it in the medical record for each patient's first office visit and electronically link it to the colonoscopy record.

DISCUSSION

The results of this scholarly project support the underlying basis for the TQM theoretical framework. Using the PDSA model, the team structure allowed stakeholders to

Table 1 Percentage and grade of endoscopic practice performance for each TQE metric						
	Documented CRC Risk Assessment	Documented Recommendations for Surveillance and Presence of Polyps	Cecal Intubation Rate	Quality of Bowel Preparation	Adenoma Detection Rate (Male/ Female)	Mean Colonoscope Withdrawal Time (Minutes)
TQE Standard	100%	100%	95%	90%	25%/15%	>6
Practice	36.7%	72.2%/83.3%	100%	91.5%	33.7%/ 30.1%	Insufficient data points
Grade	Substandard	Substandard	Met	Met	Met	Substandard

identify performance gaps, investigate root causes of deficiencies, and consider practice changes for improvement in the overall quality and effective delivery of colorectal care provided by the practice. Similarly, the findings of the project align closely with the problems in producing quality outcomes in continuous QI. The project identified supportive evidence for substandard performance that may have occurred from poor job design, failure of leadership, or an unclear purpose. It is the collective practice's responsibility to initiate QI initiatives to improve the CRC-P colonoscopy performance from outlined recommendations.

Maintaining the underlying principle of TQM (that people are basically good and work hard) allowed the stakeholders to avoid blame for or fear of the identified deficiencies. In this situation, the failure was of a system, not of individuals. Specifically, no system was in place to regularly assess endoscopists' colonoscopy performance and documentation. Thus, there was a need for QI to change the practice's systems, not criticize individual endoscopists. The stakeholders sustained respect and trust among each other and appreciated the need to be involved in the QI process.

As part of the TQM theoretical basis for this project, the stakeholders embraced the purpose for improvement in their endoscopic practice to better care for patients. Using the philosophy to improve constantly, the practice's stakeholders financially and emotionally committed a team structure to critically assess the endoscopic deficiencies in care. Problem solving by root cause analysis and identifying improvement initiatives entailed redesigning the CRC-P care processes.

Impact of Results on Practice

A transformation of health care leadership with a renewed commitment to organizational improvement is necessary to accomplish the challenge of delivering ideal care set forth by the IOM. Doctor of Nursing Practice (DNP) nurses have the leadership qualities and responsibility to impact patient care and influence patient outcomes. The DNP nurse's role in quality efforts is to reflect on and review the overall delivery of care within his or her domain of practice. The DNP nurse is obligated and accountable to ensure that the practice environment fosters the delivery of high-quality, safe, effective patient care.

Until recently, it has been assumed that the practice's endoscopists provided excellence in CRC-P given their years of training and experience. The evidence for substandard colonoscopy performance argued the converse. Conceptually, QI has been urged in the practice without an agreed on definition or designed methodology. Based on the stakeholders' commitment to providing excellence in CRC-P, they mutually understood the necessity of QI. They now agree to routinely evaluate their performance against the TQE standards and perform ongoing QI.[16]

Strengths and Limitations

Three strengths influenced the success of this project. The first strength was the theoretical framework. The TQM theory viewed the performance deficiencies as organizational issues to improve, rather than personal deficiencies of each endoscopist. This perspective prevented stakeholders from being defensive of their practice and encouraged participation in the root cause analysis for each performance gap and the practice improvement initiatives. A second strength was the methodology. The PDSA model systematically outlined the approach for measuring colonoscopy performance to identify gaps. The cycle guided the implementation of evaluating CRC-P by colonoscopy as an improvement in the real work setting. The third strength was the use of evidence-based metrics. The metrics were easily identifiable in the colonoscopy reports preventing error in the CRC-P performance measurement. Furthermore, by virtue of the metrics being evidence-based, the deficiencies identified were clearly problems relating to patient care that required remedy. The stakeholders could not dismiss these metrics as unimportant or subjective.

The acknowledged weakness is the small sample size. The review of 90 colonoscopy reports fulfilled the purpose of this study to implement an assessment of performance and develop QI initiatives. However, a larger sample would lend to a statistically significant assessment and perhaps indicate additional areas for QI. It has been noted that routine evaluations need to occur to evaluate the practice's efforts.

Recommendations for Practice

Inherent in patient care is the aim to strive for and maintain excellence. Studying individual or practice performance allows clinicians to identify gaps in quality, implement changes, and measure and report improvement. As demonstrated in this project, the PDSA model, TQM theoretical framework, and evidence-based measures are useful tools to guide clinicians to measure quality of care and improve health care delivery for favorable patient outcomes.

The realities of the health system require that clinicians also learn to thrive in an environment in which payors and patients are increasingly demanding value-based care, and reimbursement is reliant on the same. There is now an increased emphasis on how health care providers can demonstrate quality outcomes, continuous improvement, and sustained levels of excellence in the delivery of care. The use of clinical data to identify providers and practices that demonstrate quality and efficiency may impact reimbursement decisions from payors. As a result, quality measurement programs need to be implemented to provide incentives for reporting quality metrics and showing improvement.

Payors are eager to have employers and plan beneficiaries view them as fiscally responsible. For example, Medicare plans to transition reimbursement based on efficiency and the quality of services provided, instead of the quantity of services provided.[47] It is expected that payors will introduce provisions that reduce reimbursement for those who do not report their results or do not demonstrate quality sufficient to meet standards.[47] This growing interest in achieving higher-value care has led to increased efforts to improve systems for measuring care, using these measures for QI and directly linking quality outcomes to reimbursement.[47]

The demand to demonstrate and deliver quality and value of care must be a motivating factor for providers to be proactive to meet the growing expectations of consumers and payors. Well-designed and proactive monitoring of patient populations allows clinicians to actively survey and intervene as necessary to prevent adverse health events, predict patients at risk for deteriorating health, and ensure appropriate follow-up. Additionally, benchmarking outcomes provides clinicians with useful comparisons to set targets for improvement and demonstrate excellence.

SUMMARY

The needs assessment indicating the lack of evaluation of CRC-P colonoscopy performance was the impetus for this project. Implementing the measurement of colonoscopy performance and prioritizing practice improvements were a necessary change for the practice to meet the IOM dimensions of quality care.[13] The results indicated deficiencies in care to prevent CRC and initiated practice changes to better serve the practice's patient population. The success of this project was attributed to the TQM theoretical framework and the PDSA methodology. Future ongoing evaluations require a larger sample size. Regardless, this project serves as an important example to assess and improve outcomes, demonstrate gains to payors, and help the practice succeed in a value-driven health care environment.

REFERENCES

1. US Cancer Statistics Working Group. United States cancer statistics: 1999–2008 incidence and mortality web-based report. Available at: http://www.cdc.gov/uscs. Accessed May 7, 2012.
2. Hardcastle JD, Chamberlain JO, Robinson MH. Randomized controlled trial of fecal-occult blood screening for colorectal cancer. Lancet 1996;384:1472–7. http://dx.doi.org/10.1016/S0140-6736(05)62855-3.
3. Kronborg O, Fenger C, Olsen J, et al. Randomized study of screening for colorectal cancer with fecal occult blood test. Lancet 1996;348(9040):1467–71. http://dx.doi.org/10.1016/S0140-6736(96)03430-7.
4. Mandel JS, Chruch TR, Bond JH, et al. The effect of fecal occult blood screening on the incidence of colorectal cancer. N Engl J Med 2000;343:1603–7. http://dx.doi.org/10.1056/NEJMcp010886.
5. Selby JV, Friedman GD, Quesenberry CP, et al. A case-control study of screening sigmoidoscopy and mortality from colorectal cancer. N Engl J Med 1992;326(10):653–7.
6. Crowe S. Overcoming obstacles to quality measurement. AGA Perspectives 2012;8(1):2–3.
7. Levin B, Lieberman DA, McFarland B, et al. Screening and surveillance for the early detection of colorectal cancer and adenomatous polyps, 2008: a joint guideline from the American Cancer Society, the US Multi-Society Task Force on Colorectal Cancer, and the American College of Radiology. Gastroenterology 2008;134(5):1570–95. http://dx.doi.org/10.1053/j.gastro.2008.02.002.
8. Faigel DO. Proposed quality measures for CRC screening are effective. AGA Perspectives 2012;8(1):4–8.
9. Schoenfeld P. What are the benchmarks for "quality colonoscopy?". AGA Perspectives 2012;8(1):4–8.
10. American Gastroenterology Association Digestive Health Outcome Registry. Colorectal cancer prevention (CRC-P) data collection form. Available at: http://www.gastro.org/practice/digestive-health-outcomes-registry/sample-reports-forms-and-measures. Accessed July 23, 2012.
11. Camp RC, Tweet AG. Benchmarking applied to healthcare. Jt Comm J Qual Improv 1994;20(5):229–38.
12. American Gastroenterology Association Expert Panel. Colorectal cancer prevention (CRC-P) measures. Available at: http://www.gastro.org/practice/digestive-health-outcomes-registry/clinical-content/CRCprevention-measures. Accessed July 23, 2012.
13. Institute of Medicine. Crossing the quality chasm: a new health care system for the 21st century. Washington, DC: National Academy Press; 2001.
14. Radawski D. Continuous quality improvement: Origins, concepts, problems, and applications. Available at: http://www.paeaonline.org/index.php?ht=action/GetDocumentAction/i/25258. Accessed May 21, 2012.
15. Rex DK, Bond JH, Winawer S, et al, US Multi-Society Task Force on Colorectal Cancer. Quality in the technical performance of colonoscopy and the continuous quality improvement for colonoscopy: recommendations of the US Multi-Society Task Force on Colorectal Cancer. Am J Gastroenterol 2002;97(6):1296–308.

16. Rex DK, Petrini JL, Baron TH, et al. Quality indicators for colonoscopy. Gastrointest Endosc 2006;63(4):16–28.

17. Rex DK, ACG Board of Trustees. American College of Gastroenterology action plan for colorectal cancer prevention. Am J Gastroenterol 2004;99(4):574–7. http://dx.doi.org/10.1111/j.1572-0241.2004.04108.x.

18. Muller AD, Sonneberg A. Prevention of colorectal cancer by flexible endoscopy and polypectomy. A case-control study of 32,702 veterans. Ann Intern Med 1995;123(12):904–10.

19. Anderson ML, Pasha TM, Leighton JA. Endoscopic perforation of the colon: lessons from a 10-year study. Am J Gastroenterol 2000;95(12):3418–22.

20. Rex D, Cutler CS, Lemmel GT, et al. Colonoscopic miss rates of adenomas determined by back-to-back colonoscopies. Gastroenterology 1997;112(1): 24–8.

21. Waye JD, Lewis BS, Yessayan S. Colonoscopy: a prospective report of complications. J Clin Gastroenterol 1992;15(4):347–51.

22. Guyatt G, Hayward R, Richardson SW, et al. Moving from evidence to action: grading recommendations – a qualitative approach. In: Guyatt G, Rennie D, editors. Users' guides to medical literature. Chicago: AMA Press; 2002. p. 599–608.

23. Bjorkman DJ, Popp WJ. Measuring the quality of endoscopy. Gastrointest Endosc 2006;63(4):1–2. http://dx.doi.org/10.1016/j.gie.2006.02.022.

24. US Preventative Services Task Force (USPSTF). Screening for colorectal cancer: recommendation and rationale. Ann Intern Med 2000;137(2):129–31.

25. Smith RA, von Eschenbach AC, Wender R, et al. American Cancer Society guidelines for the early detection of cancer: an update of early detection guidelines for prostate, colorectal, and endometrial cancers. CA Cancer J Clin 2001;51(1): 38–71. http://dx.doi.org/10.3322/canjclin.51.1.38.

26. Winawer S, Fletcher R, Rex D, et al. Colorectal cancer screening and surveillance: clinical guidelines and rationale: update based on new evidence. Gastroenterology 2003;124(2):544–60.

27. Smith RA, Cokkinides V, von Eschenbach AC, et al. American Cancer Society guidelines for the early detection of cancer. CA: A Cancer Journal for Clinicians 2002;52(1):8–22.

28. Li J, Nadel MR, Poppell CF, et al. Quality assessment of colonoscopy reporting: results form a statewide cancer screening program. Diagn Ther Endosc 2010; 2010. http://dx.doi.org/10.1155/2010/419796.

29. Rex D, Cummings OW, Helper DJ, et al. Five year incidence of adenomas after negative colonoscopy in asymptomatic average-risk persons. Gastroenterology 1996;111(5):1178–81.

30. Newcomb PA, Storer BE, Morimoto LM, et al. Long-term efficacy of sigmoidoscopy in the reduction of colorectal cancer incidence. J Natl Cancer Inst 2003; 95(8):622–5. http://dx.doi.org/10.1093/jnci/95.8.622.

31. US Preventive Services Task Force. Screening for colorectal cancer: US Preventive Services Task Force recommendation statement. Ann Intern Med 2008; 149(9):627–37.

32. Rabeneck L, Souchek J, El-Serag HB. Survival of colorectal cancer patients hospitalized in the Veterans Affairs health care system. Am J Gastroenterol 2003; 98(11):86–92.

33. Imperiale T, Wagner D, Lin C, et al. Risk of advanced proximal neoplasms in asymptomatic adults according to the distal colorectal findings. N Engl J Med 2000;343(3):169–74.

34. US Preventive Services Task Force. US Preventative Services Task Force evidence syntheses. Available at: http://www.ncbi.nlm.nih.gov/books/NBK43437/. Accessed June 3, 2012.

35. Froelich F, Wietlisbach V, Gonvers JJ, et al. Impact of colonic cleansing on quality and diagnostic yield of colonoscopy: the European Panel of Appropriateness of Gastrointestinal Endoscopy European Multicenter Study. Gastrointest Endosc 2005;61(3):378–84. http://dx.doi.org/10.5946/ce.2012.45.2.113.

36. Harewood G, Sharma V, De Garmo P. Impact of colonoscopy preparation quality on detection of suspected colonic neoplasia. Gastrointest Endosc 2003;58(1): 76–9. http://dx.doi.org/10.1067/mge.2003.294.

37. Lieberman D, Nadel M, Smith RA, et al. Standardized colonoscopy reporting and data system: report of the quality assurance task group of the national colorectal cancer roundtable. Gastrointest Endosc 2007;65(6):757–66.

38. Lieberman D, Weiss D. VA Cooperative Study No.380 Group. One-time screening for colorectal cancer with combined fecal occult-blood test and examination of the distal colon. N Engl J Med 2001;345(8):555–60.

39. Rex D. Colonoscopic withdrawal technique is associated with adenoma miss rates. Gastrointest Endosc 2001;51(1):33–6.

40. Schoenfeld P, Cash B, Flood A, et al. Colonoscopic screening of average risk women for colorectal neoplasia. N Engl J Med 2005;352(20):2061–80.

41. Barclay RL, Vicari JJ, Doughty AS, et al. Colonoscopic withdrawal times and rates of adenoma detection during screening colonoscopy. N Engl J Med 2006;355(8): 2533–41.

42. Sanchez W, Harewood GC, Petersen BT. Evaluation of polyp detection in relation to procedure time of screening or surveillance colonoscopy. Am J Gastroenterol 2004;99(10):1941–5. http://dx.doi.org/10.1111/j.1572-0241.2004.40569.x.

43. Juran JM, Godfrey AB. Juran's quality handbook. Available at: http://www.pqmonline.com/assets/files/lib/juran.pdf. Accessed September 7, 2012.

44. Hunter DL, Kernan MT, Grubbs MR. Teamworks: a model for continuous quality improvement in the health care industry. Am J Med Qual 1995;10(4):199–205.

45. Grol R, Bosch M, Hulscher M, et al. Planning and studying improvement in patient care: the use of theoretical perspectives. Milbank Q 2007;85(1):93–138.

46. Institute for Healthcare Improvement. Plan-do-study-act (PDSA) worksheet. Available at: http://www.ihi.org/knowledge/pages/tools/plandostudyactworksheet.aspx. Accessed July 16, 2012.

47. Blum J. Improving quality, lowering costs: the role of health care delivery system. Available at: http://www.hhs.gov/asl/testify/2011/11/t20111110a.html. Accessed June 15, 2013.

Evidence-Based Protocol
Diagnosis and Treatment of Catheter-Associated Urinary Tract Infection Within Adult Neurocritical Care Patient Population

Olga Dayts, DNP, RN, ACNP-BC, CCRN

KEYWORDS

- Neurologic ICU • Urinary tract infection • Nosocomial infections
- Immunodepression syndrome

KEY POINTS

- Evidence exists that patients requiring neurologic ICU (NCU) admission have concomitant immunosuppression that makes them more prone to acquiring nosocomial infections.
- The risk of infection is highest in the acute phase after stroke, which may be attributed to stroke-induced immunodepression syndrome.
- Significant numbers of patients are being diagnosed inappropriately with catheter-associated (CA) urinary tract infection (UTI), for which they receive treatment that is not recommended.
- Protocol-based care enables providers to translate evidence into practice.

INTRODUCTION

It has been reported that admission to an NCU after stroke reduces mortality through prevention and treatment of complications, especially infection.[1] The overall clinical course of NCU patients is greatly affected, however, by the occurrence of medical complications during the course of the disease, which have a substantial impact on both mortality and long-term clinical outcome. Evidence exists that patients requiring NCU admission have concomitant immunosuppression that make them more prone to acquiring nosocomial infections.[2] The risk of infection is highest in the acute phase after stroke, which may be attributed to stroke-induced immunodepression syndrome.[3]

BACKGROUND AND SIGNIFICANCE

Recent evidence suggests that NCUs, amid all ICUs, possess a high incidence of hospital-acquired UTIs.[4,5] Therefore, strong emphasis has been recently placed on

Vanderbilt University Medical Center, 1211 Medical Center Drive, Nashville, TN 37212, USA
E-mail address: olga.dayts@vanderbilt.edu

Nurs Clin N Am 49 (2014) 29–43
http://dx.doi.org/10.1016/j.cnur.2013.11.008
0029-6465/14/$ – see front matter © 2014 Elsevier Inc. All rights reserved.

health care providers decreasing complications and improving quality across the spectrum of patient care. Beginning in October 2008, the Centers for Medicare and Medicaid Services (CMS) stopped offering additional reimbursements for patients discharged with a diagnosis of CA-UTI.[6] Among the 10 hospital-acquired conditions selected by the CMS, CA-UTI received a high priority due to its high cost and high volume.[7]

In addition, a majority of cases of nosocomial CA-UTI are really CA asymptomatic bacteriuria (CA-ASB).[8] According to the 2005 Infectious Diseases Society of America (IDSA) guidelines, CA-ASB is not a clinically significant condition, and treatment is unlikely to confer clinical benefit.[9] A significant limitation between evidence-based guidelines concerning management of CA-ASB and clinical practice has been documented, however, in recent publications from the United States, the United Kingdom, France, and Canada.[10–14] Significant numbers of patients are being diagnosed inappropriately with CA-UTI, for which they receive treatment that is not recommended. This inappropriate treatment is potentially harmful in terms of emergence of resistant pathogens, superinfections, and unnecessary costs.

PURPOSE AND SPECIFIC AIMS

Despite published guidelines for the diagnosis and optimal selection of an antimicrobial agent and duration of therapy in treating CA-UTI, NCU providers in Vanderbilt University Medical Center (VUMC) demonstrate a wide variation in its treatment practices. This may be associated with undesirable outcomes, including subsequent antimicrobial resistance, adverse drug effects, and cost. In phase 1, the purpose of this project was a quality-improvement (QI) initiative that (1) examined the prescribing practices for the treatment of CA-UTI within an NCU adult patient population, (2) determined whether these practices followed the recommendations in the IDSA guidelines, and (3) developed an evidence-based protocol for diagnosis and treatment of CA-UTI in an adult neurocritical care patient population that includes recommendations of the IDSA guidelines and the development of an NCU antibiogram. The aim of this protocol was not intended, however, to replace clinical judgment but to provide an organized method for diagnosing and treating CA-UTI within the adult neurocritical care patient population.

PRACTICE SETTING

The NCU at VUMC is a multidisciplinary 22-bed unit; 38% of the NCU patients are between the ages of 19 and 50. A majority of the patients are in the neurosurgery (56%) and neurology (29%) services. The most common 3 admitting diagnoses in the NCU are stroke (30%), seizures (15%), and brain tumors (11%). Generally, 62% of patients in NCU have a Foley catheter at some point during their admission. This NCU functions with close collaboration between multiple services; therefore, a successful protocol development within the NCU requires collaboration and commitment of all disciplines involved in providing NCU patients' care.

BENEFIT TO PRACTICE

Protocol-based care enables providers to translate evidence into practice. Protocols outline the optimal care for a specific group of patients to assist providers in making decisions regarding appropriate health care for a specific clinical situation. High-quality protocols are clear, reliable, and reproducible. Thus, they standardize practice and reduce variation in the treatment of patients, increase provider knowledge, and improve the quality of patient care.[15–18] Furthermore, it has been demonstrated that adherence to protocols may reduce health care costs up to 25%.[19] Therefore, the developed protocol for diagnosis and treatment of UTIs in the adult neurocritical care patient population can increase adherence to practice guidelines, thus improving medical management and clinical outcomes.[20] Furthermore, it has the potential to decrease length of stay, health care costs, readmission rates, complications, and resource utilization and to serve as an educational tool.[21]

CONCEPTUAL FRAMEWORK

Implementing evidence into practice requires a conceptual model that helps organize strategies and clarify variables that may influence the adoption of an evidence-based practice (EBP).[22] The Stetler model of research utilization is a practitioner-oriented model and served as the project's conceptual framework for integrating research findings into EBP. The 5 phases of the Stetler model are preparation, validation, comparative evaluation/decision making, translation/application, and evaluation.[23] Part of translation/application (phase IV) and evaluation (phase V) were not implemented, however, in the project. Thus, the phases that were implemented in the Doctor of Nursing Practice (DNP) project include

- Phase I (preparation): defining the purpose of the literature review to help in identifying evidence-based measurable outcomes; searching for applicable articles; and identifying barriers, both internal and external, that could influence the decision-making process
- Phase II (validation): critiquing the chosen literature, validating each article regarding its level of support for the topic searched and whether there is adequate evidence in the literature to continue
- Phase III (comparative evaluation/decision making): synthesizing and evaluating the evidence-based findings to determine desirability and feasibility of applying the findings to practice
- Phase IV (translation/application): translating evidence-based findings into a plan

APPRAISAL OF EVIDENCE AND SYNTHESIS

Many clinical studies were reviewed in an effort to gather evidence on diagnosis and treatment of symptomatic and asymptomatic CA-UTI.[8,9,24–42] A total of 4 IDSA guidelines were reviewed for this project, each focused on the diagnosis and treatment of 4 different types of UTIs in adults. The guidelines addressed asymptomatic bacteriuria, acute uncomplicated cystitis and pyelonephritis, symptomatic and asymptomatic CA-UTI, and urinary tract candidiasis.[24,26,43,44] This QI project only focused, however, on the diagnosis and treatment of CA-UTI in adults consistent with recommendations from the IDSA guidelines.[26] According to the IDSA guideline, "Diagnosis, Prevention, and Treatment of Catheter-Associated Urinary Tract Infection in Adults," the method of diagnosing and managing CA-UTI and CA-ASB includes the following (**Table 1**).

Needs Assessment

At the time of the DNP project, the NCU at VUMC did not have a protocol to guide clinicians in the diagnosis and management practice of CA-UTI for the NCU adult patient population. Thus, given the lack of protocol availability, the following protocol was developed. Prior to the development of an evidence-based protocol, however, a needs assessment was completed as the initial step in the beginning of the project. The analysis examined the prescribing practices for the treatment of CA-UTI within the

Table 1
Diagnosis, prevention, and treatment of catheter-associated urinary tract infection in adults

Diagnosis of CA-UTI	Treatment of CA-UTI
• CA-UTI in patients with indwelling urethral, indwelling suprapubic, or intermittent catheterization is defined by the presence of symptoms or signs compatible with UTI with no other identified source along with $\geq 10^3$ CFU/mL of 1 bacterial species in a single catheter urine specimen or in a midstream voided urine specimen from a patient whose urethral, suprapubic, or condom catheter has been removed within the previous 48 h (A-III).	• Urine specimen for culture should be obtained prior to initiating antimicrobial therapy for presumed CA-UTI due to the wide spectrum of potential infecting organisms and the increased probability of antimicrobial resistance (A-III).
• Signs and symptoms compatible with CA-UTI include new-onset or worsening of fever, rigors, altered mental status, malaise, or lethargy with no other identified cause; flank pain; costovertebral angle tenderness; acute hematuria; pelvic discomfort; and, in those whose catheters have been removed, dysuria, urgent or frequent urination, or suprapubic pain or tenderness (A-III).	• If an indwelling catheter has been in place for >2 wk at the onset of CA-UTI and still indicated, the catheter should be replaced to hasten resolution of symptoms and to reduce the risk of subsequent CA-bacteriuria and CA-UTI (A-I).
• Absence of pyuria in symptomatic patient suggests a diagnosis other than CA-UTI (A-III).	• Urine culture should be obtained from the freshly placed catheter prior to initiation of antimicrobial therapy to help guide treatment (A-II).
• In catheterized patient, presence or absence of odorous or cloudy urine alone should not be used to diagnose CA-UTI or as an indication for urine culture or antimicrobial therapy (A-III).	• If use of the catheter can be discontinued, culture of a voided midstream urine specimen should be obtained prior to initiation of antimicrobial therapy to assist guide treatment (A-III).
	• 7-Day regimen is the recommended duration of antimicrobial treatment of patients with CA-UTI who have prompt resolution of symptoms (A-III), and 10–14 d of treatment is recommended for those with a delayed response (A-III), regardless of whether the patient remains catheterized.
	• 5-Day regimen of levoflxacin may be considered in patients with CA-UTI who are not severely ill (B-III); data are insufficient to make such a recommendation about other fluoroquinolones.
	• 3-Day antimicrobial regimen may be considered for women aged ≤ 65 y who develop CA-UTI without upper urinary tract symptoms after an indwelling catheter has been removed (B-II).

Abbreviations: A, Good evidence to support the recommendation for or against use; B, Moderate evidence to support a recommendation for or against use; C, Poor evidence to support the recommendation for or against use; I, Evidence from >1 properly randomized, controlled trial; II, Evidence from >1 well-designed clinical trial, without randomization, from cohort or case-controlled analytic studies [preferably>1 center]; from multiple time-series; or from dramatic results from uncontrolled experiments; III, Evidence from opinions of respected authorities based on clinical experience, descriptive studies, or reports of expert committees.

Data from Hooton TM, Bradley SF, Cardenas DD, et al. Diagnosis, prevention, and treatment of catheter-associated urinary tract infection in adults: 2009 international clinical practice guidelines from the Infectious Diseases Society of America. Clin Infect Dis 2010;50(5):625–63.

NCU adult patient population in accordance with the IDSA guideline. Subsequently, the current practice was compared with the recommendations in the IDSA guideline. These data helped clarify the frequency of the variations in the treatment practices of CA-UTI. Hence, the purpose of this analysis was to analyze the current NCU provider treatment of CA-UTI in NCU at VUMC and determine whether these practices followed the current recommendations of the IDSA guideline.

Methodologic Framework

The purpose of this improvement project was diagnosis and management of patients in the NCU with CA-UTI within an academic medical center environment. The methodologic framework for this project's purpose was model for improvement (MFI). It directly followed and worked closely in accordance with this project's conceptual framework, the Stetler model of research utilization. The Stetler model's main goal in this project was to outline the steps in translating and integrating research findings into EBP, which were essential and must have been undertaken prior to the development of an evidence-based protocol, whereas MFI was used to further delineate and define the improvement and implementation of any new processes.

MFI guided the improvement project through iterative plan, do, study, act (PDSA) cycles. The 3 MFI questions were, What are we trying to accomplish? How will we know a change is an improvement? and What changes can we implement that will result in an improvement? The PDSA was used to describe the improvement process to further detail the MFI questions.[45]

Plan

The *plan phase* of the PDSA for the improvement effort began with a formation of a multidisciplinary work team and the development of specific aims and milestones for the improvement project. The team consisted of leaders from the NCU department of anesthesiology/division of critical care, QI, and infectious disease (ID), and ID pharmacy.

Specific aims for the plan were as follows:
- Aim 1: examine current prescribing practices for the treatment of CA-UTI within an NCU adult patient population
- Aim 2: determine whether these practices follow the recommendations in the IDSA guideline
- Aim 3: develop an evidence-based protocol for diagnosis and treatment of CA-UTI in an adult neurocritical care patient population that includes recommendations of the IDSA guideline

Measurable criteria for each of the plan's aims required the following endpoints:
- Aim 1: current prescribing practices for the treatment of CA-UTI within an NCU adult patient population have been examined.
- Aim 2: it was determined that prescribing practices did not follow the recommendations in the IDSA guideline; subsequently, data analysis was presented to stakeholders (NCU anesthesiology/critical care, QI, ID, and ID pharmacy).
- Aim 3: evidence-based protocol for diagnosis and treatment of CA-UTI in an adult neurocritical care patient population was developed that includes recommendations of the IDSA guideline; subsequently, protocol was presented to stakeholders (NCU anesthesiology/critical care, QI, ID, and ID pharmacy).

Do

The *do phase* of the PDSA described the steps of the plan phase of the PDSA model. It included operationalization of the baseline assessment of current prescribing practices for the treatment of CA-UTI within the NCU patient population and comparative analysis that determined whether these practices were consistent with the recommendations of national guidelines. In addition, it provided a description of how the baseline data and comparative analysis had an impact on the development of an evidence-based protocol for diagnosis and treatment of CA-UTI adult neurocritical care patients.

Actions for aim 1 were to
- Obtain data for all positive urine cultures in the NCU from July 2011 to June 2012. It is imperative to note that the unit of analysis for this study was a positive urine culture, classified as CA-UTI.
- Determine data elements pertinent to establishing variations in NCU provider CA-UTI treatment practices not consistent with recommendations in the IDSA guideline. The data elements that were captured by chart review include demographics (age, gender, admitting diagnosis, and day from admission to clinical signs and symptoms of CA-UTI), signs and symptoms (fever of temperature >38°C or, in those whose catheters have been removed, dysuria, urgent or frequent urination, or suprapubic pain or tenderness), present or past catheter (urethral or suprapubic) use within 48 hours, types and quantities of organisms found in the urine culture, reason for treatment of infection (if stated in the medical record), prescribed antibiotics, duration of antibiotic treatment, and type of NCU service that provided treatment. Clinical signs and symptoms, as well as specific documentation of the provider's thought process, were accepted as justification for treatment of the episode.
- Subsequently, an analytical analysis was compiled on the data obtained.

Actions for aim 2 were to
- Determine data analysis of the prescriptive practices and comparative analysis. The data analysis consisted of descriptive statistical analysis of the retrospective data noting the prescribing practices for the treatment of CA-UTI within the VUMC adult NCU patient population compared with IDSA guideline recommendations. If the prescribing practices were consistent with the IDSA guideline, they were termed, *appropriate treatment*. If the prescribing practices were not consistent with the IDSA guideline, they were labeled *divergent treatment*. Both appropriate and divergent treatments were based on classification of CA-UTI, current presence of catheter or within 48 hours, number of organisms in the urine, quantity of predominant organism in the urine, and types of organisms in the urine. Moreover, the divergent category was further subdivided into *extended treatment* or *limited treatment*. Extended treatment was defined as treatment that exceeded IDSA guideline recommendations in terms of antibiotic therapy duration. Limited treatment was defined as treatment that was less than the IDSA guideline recommendations in reference to antibiotic therapy duration.
- After the data were collected, positive urine culture was classified as CA-UTI in accordance with the definition provided in the IDSA guideline by Hooton and colleagues.[26]
- Next, the NCU provider UTI treatment practices were examined, such as the type of antibiotic prescribed and its duration of treatment, which were subsequently compared with the IDSA recommendations to determine whether the NCU providers were following the recommendations in the IDSA guideline.
- Subsequently, the data findings on whether the provider treatment of CA-UTI within the NCU patient population were consistent with the IDSA guideline were presented to the leadership from NCU anesthesiology/critical care, QI, and ID pharmacy.

Actions for aim 3 were as follows:
- Prior to establishing a protocol for the diagnosis and treatment of CA-UTI within the NCU adult patient population, input was sought from an NCU physician, ID

lead NCU physician and nurse practitioner, and ID pharmacist on individual elements that should be incorporated within an evidence-based protocol.
- Subsequently, in accordance with baseline data analysis, results of the provider prescribing practices, and input from the experts from NCU anesthesiology/critical care, ID, and ID pharmacy, protocol was developed.
- The evidence-based protocol was general, encompassing elements such as diagnostic and treatment methods of CA-UTI as recommended by the IDSA guideline, addressing the time frame on how often the NCU UTI antibiogram should be updated, emphasizing that empiric antimicrobial treatment should be tailored to the organism's culture and sensitivity results as soon as the data are available, and highlighting that the recommendations within protocol may not be appropriate for all clinical situations; thus, decisions must be based on the professional judgment of the clinician and consideration of the individual patient circumstances and available resources.

Study

The *study phase* of the PDSA involved an analysis of how the aims were to be carried out from the plan phase of the PDSA model. It consisted of quantitative analysis of prescribing practices for the treatment of CA-UTI and comparative analysis of these practices to the recommendations of the IDSA guideline to determine whether these practices followed the recommendations of national guidelines. Quantitative analysis was essential for the development of an evidence-based protocol, which was developed.

Act

The *act phase* of the PDSA typically consists of an implementation and dissemination of an improvement. Essential to this phase was the development of an evidence-based protocol for diagnosis and treatment of CA-UTI within the adult NCU patient population. In order to attain stakeholder buy-in of the protocol, an organizational leadership meeting will be scheduled in phase 2 of this project, where an evidence-based protocol will be presented to the director of the NCU and leaders in ID, QI, and ID pharmacy. Organizational leadership approval is essential to the success of the implementation and dissemination of the protocol. It ensures that the leadership team supports the efforts put forth into the development of the protocol, thus understanding and accepting the protocol during its implementation and dissemination process.

PROJECT RESULTS

Demographic data of patients with CA-UTI in NCU at VUMC over a 12-month period were analyzed (**Table 2**). Treatment of CA-UTI in NCU at VUMC over a 12-month period was examined (**Table 3**). Data elements of patients pertinent to diagnosis of CA-UTI in NCU at VUMC over a 12-month period were collected (**Table 4**). Evidence-Based Protocol: Diagnosis and Treatment of Catheter Associated Urinary Tract Infection within Adult Neurocritical Care Patient Population was developed (**Box 1**).

Discussion of Project Results

The project results support its conceptual and methodologic framework as well as its aims and objectives. The development of an evidence-based protocol was accomplished by following the groundwork of both conceptual and methodologic frameworks, which outlined step-by step processes in translating and integrating research findings into EBP as well as delineating and defining the improvement and implementation of new processes. Furthermore, the project results revealed that the variation in

Table 2
Demographic data of patients with CA-UTI in NCU at VUMC over a 12-month period

CA-UTI	Total (n = 40)
Gender	
Female	26 (65)
Male	14 (35)
Age[a]	31–85
Day from admission to signs/symptoms of CA-UTI	
Female	8.5
Male	6.4
Admitting diagnosis	
Intracranial hemorrhage[b]	18 (45)
Ischemic cerebrovascular accident	7 (17.5)
Seizures	5 (12.5)
Spine surgery	4 (10)
Altered mental status	2 (5)
Craniotomy	1 (2.5)
Hydrocephalus	1 (2.5)
Myasthenia gravis	1 (2.5)
Hypoxia	1 (2.5)

Note: data are no. (%) of patients.
[a] Range of years.
[b] Intraparenchymal hemorrhage, intraventricular hemorrhage, or subdural hematoma.

Table 3
Treatment of CA-UTI in NCU at VUMC over a 12-month period

CA-UTI	Total (n = 40)
Appropriate treatment	28 (70)
Critical care	27 (96.4)
Neurology	1 (3.6)
Neurosurgery	0
Divergent treatment	12 (30)
Extended treatment	1 (8.3)
Critical care	1 (8.3)
Neurology	0
Neurosurgery	0
Limited treatment	11 (91.7)
Critical care	7 (63.6)
Neurology	3 (27.3)
Neurosurgery	1 (9.1)

Note: data are no. (%) of patients.

Table 4
Data elements pertinent in establishing diagnosis of CA-UTI in NCU at VUMC over a 12-month period

CA-UTI	Total (n = 40)
Catheter	
Foley catheter[a]	39 (97.5)
Suprapubic catheter	1 (2.5)
Signs/symptoms	
Fever[b]	37 (92.5)
Dysuria, urgent/frequent urination, suprapubic pain/tenderness	3 (7.5)

Organism/Quantity	Total (n = 44)	10–25 K	15–50 K	25–50 K	50–100 K	>100 K
Escherichia coli	11 (25)	0	0	2 (18.2)	2 (18.2)	7 (63.6)
Klebsiella pneumoniae	9 (20.5)	1 (11.1)	0	0	1 (11.1)	7 (77.8)
Enterococcus faecalis	7 (15.9)	1 (14.3)	0	0	0	6 (85.7)
Pseudomonas aeruginosa	4 (9.1)	1 (25)	0	2 (50)	0	1 (25)
Enterobacter cloacae	2 (4.5)	0	0	2 (100)	0	0
Enterococcus faecium	1 (2.3)	0	0	0	0	1 (100)
Escherichia coli ESBL	1 (2.3)	0	0	0	0	1 (100)
Citrobacter werkmanii	1 (2.3)	0	1 (100)	0	0	0
Proteus mirabilis	1 (2.3)	0	0	0	0	1 (100)
Streptococcus agalactiae	1 (2.3)	0	0	0	0	1 (100)

Antibiotic/Duration	Total (n = 44)	3 d	5 d	6 d	7 d	10 d
Levaquin	9 (22.5)	1	6	0	2	0
Macrobid	6 (15)	0	1	0	5	0
Ciprofloxacin	6 (15)	1	11	0	2	1
Zosyn	4 (10)	0	1	0	3	0
Bactrim	3 (7.5)	1	1	0	1	0
Cefepime	2 (5)	0	0	1	1	0
Meropenem	1 (2.5)	0	0	0	1	0
Vancomycin, Zosyn	6 (15)	1	0	0	5	0
Vancomycin, Doripenem	1 (2.5)	0	0	0	1	0
Vancomycin, Levaquin	1 (2.5)	0	0	0	1	0
Vancomycin, Cefepime	1 (2.5)	0	0	0	1	0

Note: data are no. (%) of patients.
Abbreviation: ESBL, extended-spectrum β-lactamase.
[a] Present or past catheter use within 48 hours.
[b] Fever is temperature >38°C.

prescribing practices for the treatment of CA-UTI within an adult NCU patient population showed that provider practices are not consistent with the recommendations of the IDSA guideline because 30% of patients with CA-UTI were treated divergently from recommendations of national guidelines. Therefore, evidence-based protocols need to be developed to standardize practice in diagnosis and treatment of CA-UTI. Furthermore, the development of evidence-based protocol set the stage for clinical research to determine if this DNP project will improve patient outcomes, decrease antimicrobial resistance, and reduce health care costs.

Box 1
Evidence-based protocol: diagnosis and treatment of catheter-associated urinary tract infection within an adult neurocritical care patient population

I. Population

In-hospital, with emphasis on the care of adult neurocritical care patients

II. Indications

This evidence-based protocol provides diagnostic criteria and management strategies for patients with symptomatic CA-UTI. It is intended for use by health care providers who perform direct patient care.

III. Diagnostic criteria

- CA-UTI is defined in patients with indwelling urethral, indwelling suprapubic, or intermittent catheterization with presence of symptoms or signs compatible with UTI with no other identified source of infection along with $\geq 10^3$ colony-forming units (CFU)/mL of ≥ 1 bacterial species in a single catheter urine specimen or in a midstream voided urine specimen from a patient whose urethral, suprapubic, or condom catheter has been removed within the previous 48 hours.
  - Data are inadequate to recommend a specific quantitative count for defining CA-UTI in symptomatic men when specimens are collected by condom catheter.
- Signs and symptoms compatible with CA-UTI include new-onset or worsening of fever (>38°C), rigors, altered mental status, malaise, or lethargy with no other identified cause; flank pain; costovertebral angle tenderness; acute hematuria; pelvic discomfort; and, in those whose catheters have been removed, dysuria, urgent or frequent urination, or suprapubic pain or tenderness
  - In patients with spinal cord injury, increased spasticity, autonomic dysreflexia, or sense of unease
- In catheterized patients, pyuria is *NOT* diagnostic of CA-UTI.
  - The absence of pyuria in symptomatic patients suggests a diagnosis other than CA-UTI.
- In catheterized patients, absence of odorous or cloudy urine alone should *NOT* be used to diagnose CA-UTI or as an indication for urine culture or antimicrobial therapy.

IV. Management strategies

- A urine specimen for culture should be obtained prior to initiating antimicrobial therapy for presumed CA-UTI due to the wide spectrum of potential infecting organisms and the increased probability of antimicrobial resistance.
- If an indwelling catheter has been in place for >2 weeks at the onset of CA-UTI and is still indicated, the catheter should be replaced to hasten resolution of symptoms and to reduce the risk of subsequent CA-UTI.
  - The urine culture should be obtained from the freshly placed catheter prior to the initiation of antimicrobial therapy to help guide treatment.
  - If use of the catheter can be discontinued, a culture of a voided midstream urine specimen should be obtained prior to the initiation of antimicrobial therapy to assist guide treatment.
- Empiric antimicrobial treatment should be selected according to an NCU antibiogram and tailored to an organism's culture and sensitivity results as soon as the data are available.
  - Antibiogram should be constructed and updated annually in order to provide clinicians with useful data regarding selection of appropriate empiric antimicrobial therapy.
- A 7-day regimen is the recommended duration of antimicrobial treatment of patients with CA-UTI who have prompt resolution of symptoms, and 10–14 days of treatment is recommended for those with a delayed response, regardless of whether a patient remains catheterized.

○ A 5-day regimen of levofloxacin may be considered in patients with CA-UTI who are not severely ill. Data are insufficient to make such a recommendation about other fluoroquinolones.

○ A 3-day antimicrobial regimen may be considered for women ages ≤65 years who develop CA-UTI without upper urinary tract symptoms after an indwelling catheter has been removed.

○ For patients with spinal cord injury, treatment of CA-UTI for 14 days is recommended because it leads to improved clinical and microbiological outcomes compared with short-course therapy.

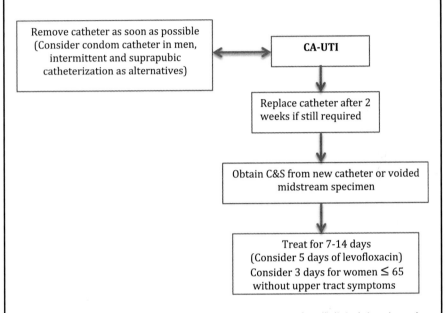

The recommendations within protocol may not be appropriate for all clinical situations; thus, decisions must be based on professional judgment of a clinician, consideration of patient circumstances, and available resources.

Abbreviation: C&S, culture and sensitivity.
From Hooton TM, Bradley SF, Cardenas DD, et al. Diagnosis, prevention, and treatment of catheter-associated urinary tract infection in adults: 2009 international clinical practice guidelines from the Infectious Diseases Society of America. Clin Infect Dis 2010;50:625–63; with permission.

Strengths and Limitations of Project

The project's overall strength consists of data analysis of provider practices, which disclosed that NCU prescriber practices in treatment of CA-UTI are not consistent with the recommendations of national guidelines, which set the platform for protocol development to standardize diagnosis and treatment of CA-UTI in neurocritical care patient populations that should be geared toward the critical care team. The project possesses several limitations, however. The first limitation of the project consists of the performance of retrospective data analysis because it relies on accuracy of the written record, thus may institute bias. The second limitation comprises inability to use an exact definition of CA-UTI according to the IDSA guidelines in the neurocritical care patient population, thus allowing room for misdiagnosis of CA-UTI in patients who are neurocritically ill. The third limitation consists of the small sample size, which comprised 40 incidences of CA-UTI that were used to examine the prescribing practices, which they may not sufficiently represent an entire NCU patient population. Furthermore, it may contain less external validity and might perhaps lead to an inappropriate generalization regarding provider treatment practices.

Dissemination of Project

After the protocol is approved by the experts in the fields of neurocritical care, ID, clinical pharmacology, and QI, the protocol will be presented to the director of the NCU for review and feedback. Once approved, it will be disseminated to other services involved in the care of the NCU patients. On approval of all the services, such as neurology, neurosurgery, and critical care, it will be implemented within the NCU. Furthermore, after implementation of protocol in the NCU, it can be modified for other patient populations and disseminated to various other specialty units within VUMC to standardize providers' practices in diagnosis and treatment of CA-UTI according to the recommendations of the national guidelines.

Future Direction of Project

In phase 1 of this project, the goal was to learn and practice the process of developing an EBP protocol. Thus, this phase consisted of an evidence appraisal for CA-UTI, which set the stage for an algorithmic approach to both CA-UTI and CA-ASB. Because improvement is about iterative cycles and small tests of change, the proof of concept was done on CA-UTI first and will be expanded to CA-ASB. In phase 2 of this project, an iterative PDSA approach will be used and future studies will address the diagnosis and management of CA-ASB in an NCU patient population. In addition, an ultimate goal of future studies will be to develop a provider resource tool, such as a pocket card that outlines the major points in diagnostic and treatment methods of both CA-UTI and CA-ASB.

This QI initiative supports the nationwide efforts to move advancements in science from bench to bedside. Translating research into clinical practice is challenging for staff across many disciplines; however, developing evidence-based protocols may facilitate the adoption of evidence-based medicine within health care organizations. Such endeavors are vital to the future of medicine.[46]

REFERENCES

1. Govan L, Langhorne P, Weir CJ. Does the prevention of complications explain the survival benefit of organized inpatient (stroke unit) care? Further analysis of a systematic review. Stroke 2007;38:2536–40.
2. Zolldann D, Spitzer C, Hafner H, et al. Surveillance of nosocomial Infections in a neurologic intensive care unit. Infect Control Hosp Epidemiol 2005;26:726–31.
3. Wartenberg KE, Stoll A, Funk A, et al. Infection after acute ischemic stroke: risk factors, biomarkers, and outcome. Stroke Res Treat 2011;830614:1–8.
4. Di Filippo A, Casini A, de Gaudio AR. Infection prevention in the intensive care unit: review of the recent literature on the management of invasive devices. Scand J Infect Dis 2011;43:243–50.
5. Gastmeier P, Behnke M, Schwab F, et al. Benchmarking of urinary tract infection rates: experiences from the intensive care unit component of the German national nosocomial infection surveillance system. J Hosp Infect 2011;78:41–4.

6. Wald HL, Kramer AM. Nonpayment for hams resulting from medical care: catheter-associated urinary tract infections. JAMA 2007;298:2782–4.
7. Titsworth WL, Hester J, Correira T, et al. Reduction of catheter-associated urinary tract infections among patients in a neurological intensive care unit: a single institution's success. J Neurosurg 2012;116:911–20.
8. Tambyah PA, Maki DG. The relationship between pyuria and infection in patients with indwelling urinary catheters: a prospective study of 761 patients. Arch Intern Med 2000;160:673–7.
9. Nicolle LE. Catheter-related urinary tract infection. Drugs Aging 2005;22:627–39.
10. Bonnal C, Baune B, Mion M, et al. Bacteriuria in a geriatric hospital: impact of an antibiotic improvement program. J Am Med Dir Assoc 2008;9:605–9.
11. Cope M, Cevallos ME, Cadle RM, et al. Inappropriate treatment of catheter-associated asymptomatic bacteriuria in a tertiary care hospital. Clin Infect Dis 2009;48:1182–8.
12. Dalen DM, Zvonar RK, Jessamine PG. An evaluation of the management of asymptomatic catheter-associated bacteriuria and candiduria at The Ottawa Hospital. Can J Infect Dis Med Microbiol 2005;16:166–70.
13. Gross PA, Patel B. Reducing antibiotic overuse: a call for a national performance measure for not treating asymptomatic bacteriuria. Clin Infect Dis 2007;45:1335–7.
14. Woodford HJ, George J. Diagnosis and management of urinary tract infection in hospitalized older people. J Am Geriatr Soc 2009;57:107–14.
15. Gawande A. The checklist manifesto: how to get things right. New York: Metropolitan Books; 2009.
16. Kirkpatrick DH, Burkman RT. Does standardization of care through clinical guidelines improve outcomes and reduce medical liability? Obstet Gynecol 2010;116:1022–6.
17. Berwick DM. A user's manual for the IOM's 'Quality Chasm' report. Health Aff (Millwood) 2002;21:80–90.
18. Grol R. Between evidence-based practice and total quality management: the implementation of cost-effective care. Int J Qual Health Care 2000;12:297–304.
19. Clayton P, Hripsak G. Decision support in healthcare. Int J Biomed Comput 1995;39:59–66.
20. Diederik WJ, Simoons D, Simoons ML. Improving adherence to guidelines for acute stroke management. Circulation 2009;119:16–8.
21. Delaney CP, Fazio VW, Senagore AJ, et al. 'Fast track' postoperative management protocol for patients with high co-morbidity undergoing complex abdominal and pelvic colorectal surgery. Br J Surg 2002;88:1533–8.
22. Titler M. Translating research into practice. Am J Nurs 2007;107:26–33.
23. Stetler CB. Updating the Stetler model of research utilization to facilitate evidence-based practice. Nurs Outlook 2001;49:272–9.
24. Nicolle LE, Bradley S, Colgan R, et al. Infectious diseases society of america guidelines for the diagnosis and treatment of asymptomatic bacteriuria in adults. Clin Infect Dis 2005;40:643–54.
25. Gould CV, Umscheid CA, Agarwal RK, et al. Guideline for prevention of catheter-associated urinary tract infections 2009. Infect Control Hosp Epidemiol 2010;31:319–26.
26. Hooton TM, Bradley SF, Cardenas DD, et al. Diagnosis, prevention, and treatment of catheter-associated urinary tract infection in adults: 2009 International Clinical Practice Guidelines from the Infectious Diseases Society of America. Clin Infect Dis 2010;50:625–63.

27. Horan TC, Andrus M, Dudeck MA. CDC/NHSN surveillance definition of health care-associated infection and criteria for specific types of infections in the acute care setting. Am J Infect Control 2010;36:309–32.
28. Trautner BW. Management of Catheter-Associated Urinary Tract Infection (CAUTI). Curr Opin Infect Dis 2010;23:76–82.
29. Nicolle LE. A practical guide to antimicrobial management of complicated urinary tract infection. Drugs Aging 2001;18:243–54.
30. Raz R, Schiller D, Nicolle LE. Chronic indwelling catheter replacement before antimicrobial therapy for symptomatic urinary tract infection. J Urol 2000;164:1254–8.
31. Bergqvist D, Bronnestam R, Hedelin H, et al. The relevance of urinary sampling methods in patients with indwelling Foley catheters. Br J Urol 1980;52:92–5.
32. Grahn D, Norman DC, White ML, et al. Validity of urinary catheter specimen for diagnosis of urinary tract infection in the elderly. Arch Intern Med 1985;145:1858–60.
33. Tenney JH, Warren JW. Bacteriuria in women with long-term catheters: paired comparison of indwelling and replacement catheters. J Infect Dis 1988;157:199–202.
34. Schwartz DS, Barone JE. Correlation of urinalysis and dipstick results with catheter-associated urinary tract infections in surgical ICU patients. Intensive Care Med 2006;32:1797–801.
35. Norberg B, Norberg A, Parkhede U, et al. Effect of short-term high- dose treatment with methenamine hippurate on urinary infection in geriatric patients with an indwelling catheter. IV. Eur J Clin Pharmacol 1979;15:357–61.
36. Walker S, McGeer A, Simor AE, et al. Why are antibiotics prescribed for asymptomatic bacteriuria in institutionalized elderly people? A qualitative study of physicians' and nurses' perceptions. CMAJ 2000;163:273–7.
37. Nicolle LE. Consequences of asymptomatic bacteriuria in the elderly. Int J Antimicrob Agents 1994;4:107–11.
38. Nicolle LE. Urinary tract infections in long-term-care facilities. Infect Control Hosp Epidemiol 2001;22:167–75.
39. Warren JW. Catheter-associated bacteriuria in long-term care facilities. Infect Control Hosp Epidemiol 1994;15:557–62.
40. Stamm WE, Hooton TM. Management of urinary tract infections in adults. N Engl J Med 1993;329:1328–34.
41. Harding GK, Nicolle LE, Ronald AR, et al. How long should catheter-acquired urinary tract infection in women be treated? A randomized, controlled study. Ann Intern Med 1991;114:713–9.
42. Peterson J, Kaul S, Khashab M, et al. A double-blind, randomized comparison of levofloxacin 750 mg once-daily for five days with ciprofloxacin 400/500 mg twice-daily for 10 days for the treatment of complicated urinary tract infections and acute pyelonephritis. Urology 2008;71:17–22.
43. Gupta K, Hooton TM, Naber KG, et al. International clinical practice guidelines for the treatment of acute uncomplicated cystitis and pyelonephritis in women: a 2010 update by the Infectious Diseases Society of America and the European Society of Microbiology and Infectious Diseases. Clin Infect Dis 2011;52:e103–20.
44. Pappas PG, Kauffman CA, Andres D, et al. Clinical practice guidelines for the management of candidiasis: 2009 update by the Infectious Diseases Society of America. Clin Infect Dis 2009;48:503–35.

45. Institute for Healthcare Improvement. How to improve. 2011. Available at: http://www.ihi.org/knowledge/Pages/HowtoImprove/default.aspx. Accessed October 10, 2012.

46. Schulman C. Strategies for starting a successful evidence-based practice program. AACN Adv Crit Care 2008;19:301–11.

Using Dedicated Nurses to Improve Core Measures Compliance

Amanda Green, DNP, RN, Lacey Buckler, DNP, RN, ACNP-BC, NE-BC*

KEYWORDS

- Core measures • Nursing • Standard work • The Joint Commission

KEY POINTS

- Quality outcomes are the focus of today's health care.
- Using a multidisciplinary team to review the process, issues, and solutions is important for success.
- Nurses dedicated to focusing on core measures increase and sustain compliance.

INTRODUCTION

Modern health care has become much more focused on tracking quality outcomes and creating transparent standards of care for hospitals compliance. Although clinicians have always endeavored to provide the best care for every patient every time, with the change in the health care climate to avoid reimbursement penalties, a focus on effectiveness and efficiency continues to be a must. Overall, the gains in performance metrics have been slow and inconsistent, with hospitals providing sophisticated and exceptional health care yet with varying quality, lack of adherence to evidence-based practice, and an accelerated cost.[1]

To encourage adoption of evidence-based guidelines, The Joint Commission (TJC) sought to build a set of metrics for 4 common diagnoses that would be the initial core measures released in 2001. By 2002, after collaboration with Centers for Medicare & Medicaid (CMS) and other key stakeholders, the first data submission was required by participating hospitals to score their compliance.[2] As of 2004, CMS produced their starter set of 10 metrics. These inpatient metrics have evolved to currently include acute myocardial infarction (AMI), heart failure (HF), pneumonia, surgical care improvement project (SCIP), childhood asthma care, stroke, immunizations, emergency department metrics, inpatient psychiatric services, and perinatal care.[3]

University of Kentucky HealthCare, Office of Enterprise Quality and Safety, 800 Rose Street, Lexington, KY 40536, USA
* Corresponding author.
E-mail address: latrou0@email.uky.edu

Nurs Clin N Am 49 (2014) 45–51
http://dx.doi.org/10.1016/j.cnur.2013.11.001
0029-6465/14/$ – see front matter © 2014 Elsevier Inc. All rights reserved.

Compliance with these national benchmarks not only represented a piece of the TJC accreditation process but also began to be publicly reported for patients to view.[4]

PROBLEM

Like many other comparable academic medical centers, the University of Kentucky Healthcare (UKHC) system was also struggling to meet the metrics with 100% compliance. The first issue encountered by the clinical leaders in service lines that have large volumes of core measure applicable patients was the lack of knowledge of performance. Before the initiation of a system-level focus on these metrics, the data were housed in the quality department, which had a limited partnership with the clinicians. The first important step to success was a link between these groups that functioned as a working partnership. Having transparent knowledge of the performance and engaging nurse and physician leadership led to a platform for investigating system-wide solutions.

DISCUSSION

First, it was necessary to determine the opportunities of missed patient care to improve core measure performance. A multidisciplinary team consisting of physicians, advanced practice providers, nurses, and pharmacists reviewed each missed opportunity and found it was necessary to first identify these core measure–eligible patients concurrently during hospitalization. To do this, the team collaborated with nurse informaticists to develop a process of identifying these patients within the electronic medical record. An order was created that identified the patient as a potential core measures candidate for HF, pneumonia, stroke, or AMI. All physicians, advanced practice providers, and nurses within the organization had the ability to submit this order on a patient. Nurses within the quality department who specialized in core measures also reviewed patients each day to identify potential patients. When this order was submitted on a patient, an icon also appeared in the patient's electronic record beside the patient's name so that bedside clinicians could easily identify them and perform appropriate care. This identification process within the medical record proved to be a valuable step in identifying these patients during hospitalization. However, this process did not completely resolve all of the missed opportunities.

Further analysis of missed opportunities showed that it was necessary to develop a team of clinicians to daily monitor these patients. It was determined that nurses would be best able to review the patients and work with the health care team daily to improve the quality of care provided. A group of 6 nurses was identified and a pilot program was initiated. Initially these nurses began monitoring patients with HF because this population historically had the largest opportunity for improvement. The nurses monitored these patients daily to confirm that heart failure teaching was completed and that an ejection fraction (EF) was either documented or planned. They also received an alert before the discharge of each identified patient. Before the patient was discharged, the nurse reviewed the discharge instructions to ensure that the patient had a complete list of discharge medications and a follow-up appointment. For patients with left ventricular systolic dysfunction, the nurse also reviewed the medication list to make sure that an angiotensin-converting enzyme inhibitor (ACEI) or angiotensin receptor blocker (ARB) medication was ordered. The nurses contacted the providers caring for the patient as necessary so that each of these components was completed before the patient was discharged. The bedside clinicians caring for the patients were aware of this review and did not allow the patient to leave the facility until the review had been completed. The monitoring of these patients by nurses proved to be successful, and compliance immediately improved for patients with HF.

Based on the success of using nurses to improve performance with the heart failure metric, the scope of these nurses was expanded to include monitoring of other core measures, including patients with AMI and pneumonia. These nurses monitored patients with AMI starting on the day of admission for compliance with the measure related to an aspirin (ASA) being given within 24 hours of admission. If an aspirin was not ordered or was ordered but had not been given, the nurse contacted the appropriate provider. These patients were also monitored at discharge to ensure that an aspirin, β-blockers, and statin medication were included on the discharge medication list. Patients with pneumonia were also monitored to verify that a blood culture was drawn when necessary and that the appropriate antibiotics were ordered and received in a timely fashion. The nurses also contacted the providers caring for these patients when necessary. Performance on these 2 core measure sets also improved substantially after the implementation of monitoring by these nurses.

Further use of these nurses to improve the quality of care provided to patients extended to those being treated for strokes and those undergoing surgical procedures. Patients treated for strokes were monitored on the day of admission to verify that the appropriate venous thromboembolism prophylaxis and antithrombotic therapy was being administered. The patients were monitored throughout the hospitalization to ensure that stroke teaching was provided and that the need for rehabilitation services was addressed. On discharge, the nurses verified that the discharge medication list was complete. The list was also reviewed to verify that antithrombotic and statin medications were ordered as appropriate.

Improving patient outcomes related to patients undergoing surgical procedures was a slightly more challenging task. To do this, the nurses had to monitor all operating room (OR) cases throughout the day to recognize those included in the SCIP. The nurses had access to the OR patient status board and monitored it throughout the day, and also ran a report each morning to review overnight cases. When surgery was completed on each patient with a procedure included in SCIP, the nurses would go to the floor where the patient was located and review the chart. The nurses monitored antibiotic use and timing during the procedure through a review of the paper anesthesia record. On postoperative days 1 and 2, the nurses monitored for antibiotic, Foley catheter, and β-blockers use as appropriate. The nurses would contact the providers caring for the patient when antibiotics were extended to verify appropriate use. The nurse would also contact the team when β-blockers were not reordered after surgery to ensure compliance. Finally, the nurses also monitored for Foley catheter use to ensure that the organization's urinary catheter protocol was being implemented appropriately.

In addition to monitoring for diagnosis-specific core measures, these nurses also followed patients for the global measures, including immunizations. The nurses would review the screening for each patient identified for a diagnosis-specific core measure to ensure that appropriate screening had been completed. If screening was not completed, the nurse would contact the provider to assist as necessary. Other global measures monitored included the tobacco treatment and substance use measure. The nurses received training in brief intervention skills and provided brief interventions as appropriate to patients with unhealthy alcohol use. The nurses also worked with the health care team to schedule outpatient referrals for substance use counseling for patients who requested these. Finally, the nurses compiled a list of patients who needed to receive follow-up phone calls to discuss tobacco, alcohol, or drug use after discharge. This list was then sent to the organization's call center that was responsible for performing these follow-up phone calls.

Initially the nurses completed all of this monitoring through the use of a paper checklist. **Fig. 1** is a portion of the checklist. All of the measures were compiled into one checklist that was used for each patient and kept in a centralized location. However, the necessity for a form within the electronic medical record was soon realized, and nurse informaticists worked with the team to develop this. This form was available for the nurses participating in the pilot to complete. Only these nurses had rights to create and modify this document. However, any clinician could review this note to determine core measure compliance. Because the organization is composed of 2 hospitals, this note has been very useful for patients who are transferred between the facilities. The note has also been beneficial to abstractors who review the charts after discharge and prepare the chart for submission.

Based on the success of this pilot program, it was determined that the need for these nurses necessitated permanent positions. Six nurses were hired into the roles on a permanent basis with the title of Clinical Quality Specialists. These nurses provided coverage 7 days a week and were in the hospital for 12 hours daily. The nurses also provided coverage for both hospitals located within the organization. These nurses followed a daily standard work guide to ensure that the same monitoring was completed each day, regardless of the nurse working. **Fig. 2** illustrates the daily standard work followed by the clinical quality specialists. This standard work is revised frequently because of the rapidly changing world of core measures. As measures are introduced and retired and manual processes are automated within the system, the standard work is also updated.

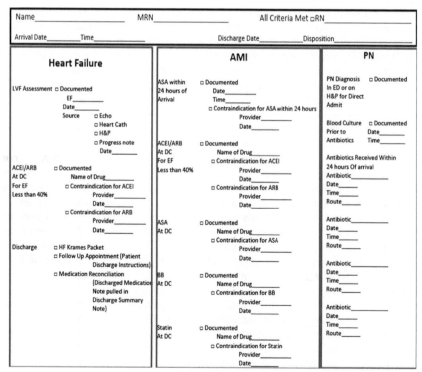

Fig. 1. Portion of the global core measures checklist for nurses. LVF, Left Ventricular Function.

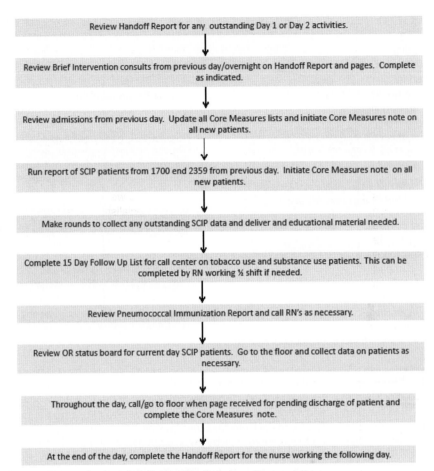

Review Handoff Report for any outstanding Day 1 or Day 2 activities.

Review Brief Intervention consults from previous day/overnight on Handoff Report and pages. Complete as indicated.

Review admissions from previous day. Update all Core Measures lists and initiate Core Measures note on all new patients.

Run report of SCIP patients from 1700 end 2359 from previous day. Initiate Core Measures note on all new patients.

Make rounds to collect any outstanding SCIP data and deliver and educational material needed.

Complete 15 Day Follow Up List for call center on tobacco use and substance use patients. This can be completed by RN working ½ shift if needed.

Review Pneumococcal Immunization Report and call RN's as necessary.

Review OR status board for current day SCIP patients. Go to the floor and collect data on patients as necessary.

Throughout the day, call/go to floor when page received for pending discharge of patient and complete the Core Measures note.

At the end of the day, complete the Handoff Report for the nurse working the following day.

Fig. 2. Daily standard work followed by clinical quality specialists.

In addition to monitoring for core measures compliance, the nurses also made rounds on the floors to work with the bedside clinicians. Each nurse was assigned units on which to make weekly rounds. Through having assigned units for each nurse, relationships were able to be built between the clinical quality specialists and the bedside clinicians. This relationship with the bedside clinicians has been beneficial in helping to educate about the importance of core measures in improving patient outcomes. The clinical quality specialists had a strong focus on educating clinicians on the evidence that supported each measure, and worked to ensure that all health care providers understand the improved patient outcomes that result from compliance with core measures.

To assist with the education for the clinicians, a standard work document for each measure set was created. This document clearly delineated the responsibilities of both the physician or advanced practice provider and the nurse. A binder with each of these documents was given to each unit to be kept at the nurses' desk. Clinicians were able to review these documents any time a question arose concerning measures applicable for a patient. **Fig. 3** is an example of the standard work for patients with HF.

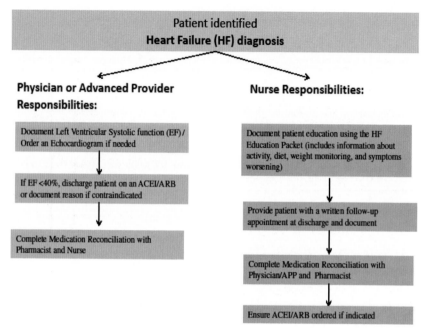

Fig. 3. Standard work for patients with HF.

The future goal is for the clinical quality specialists to continue to expand their scope. For example, the organization currently participates in the Children's Asthma Care core measures, and work is underway for these nurses to play a part in monitoring those patients. The Perinatal Core Measures will also be required by TJC starting in January 2014, and these nurses will be involved in monitoring those measures. Finally, the clinical quality specialists will also play a key role in monitoring all patients for the global core measures, such as venous thromboembolism and immunizations. Although these nurses have helped monitor these measures on patients already identified for a diagnosis-specific measure set, they are currently not monitoring all patients throughout the organization.

To monitor all patients within the organization for the global core measures, the team has been working with nurse informaticists to develop reports from within the electronic medical record to help monitor measures that have opportunity for improvement. One of these opportunities involves ensuring that sequential compression devices (SCDs) are documented as applied on all patients with an order for them. To do this, a report has been built that shows all patients who have an order for SCDs and no documentation that they were either applied or refused by the patient. The clinical quality specialists will be able to use this report to communicate with the bedside clinician to ensure that the patients are receiving quality care and that it is documented appropriately.

SUMMARY

Developing and implementing the role of these nurses has proven to be immensely valuable to the health care system. Initial tracking of these metrics can be seen in **Fig. 4**. The core measures nurses were implemented in the fourth quarter of 2011.

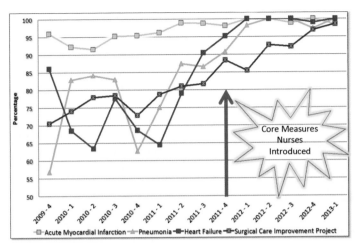

Fig. 4. UKHC core measures performance trends.

At that point, a dramatic increase in compliance occurred to near perfection, with sustained success. Prompt intervention, standard work, concurrent review, and optimization of the electronic clinical documentation were all strategies these nurses used to ensure compliance.[1] Increased awareness and transparency of the system performance has also led to a culture of accountability as a result of the intervention. Using a nurse to function in this quality role was somewhat novel to the institution but has shown success. With multiple future quality metrics on the horizon, these roles will continue to be valuable to the organization. Through focusing on core measures perfection and deploying resources for attainment, UKHC is poised to have continued success.

REFERENCES

1. Perlin J, Horner S, Englebright J, et al. Rapid core measure improvement through a "business case for quality". J Healthc Qual 2012. [Epub ahead of print].
2. Core measure sets. The Joint Commission Web site. Available at: http://www.jointcommission.org/core_measure_sets.aspx. Accessed October 20, 2013.
3. A blueprint for the CMS Measures Management System. Centers for Medicare & Medicaid Services Web site. Available at: http://www.jointcommission.org/core_measure_sets.aspx. Accessed October 20, 2013.
4. Hill PM, Rothman R, Saheed M, et al. A comprehensive approach to achieving near 100% compliance with the Joint Commission Core Measures for pneumonia antibiotic timing. Am J Emerg Med 2011;29:989–98.

Pain, Perceptions, and Perceived Conflicts: Improving the Patient's Experience

Patricia Kunz Howard, PhD, RN, CEN, CPEN, NE-BC, FAEN, FAAN[a],*,
Penne Allison, RN, BSN, MSOM, NE-BC[b], Matthew Proud, BSN, RN, CEN[c],
Jennifer Forman, RN, BSN[d]

KEYWORDS

- Pain • Perceptions • Patient • Experience • Clinical outcomes • Management

KEY POINTS

- Provider attitudes about pain management may influence the patient's feelings about their care in the emergency department.
- There is support that patients' perceptions of their care, and specifically management of their pain, impacts their clinical outcomes.
- Pain education and innovative approaches to nurse-driven protocols are essential to ensure the most optimal provision of care and clinical outcomes.

INTRODUCTION

Pain is the number 1 reason patients 15 years of age and older seek care in an emergency department (ED).[1] ED visits for nontraumatic abdominal pain increased 31% from 1999 to 2008.[1] Patients' experiences with pain management in the ED may be impacted most by delays in crowded emergency departments. Provider attitudes about pain management may influence patients' feelings about their care in the ED. Innovative strategies for pain management need to be considered to meet patients' expectations about their pain.

BACKGROUND

A review of the literature provides substantive evidence that pain management in the ED does not meet patients' expectations of care related to their pain.[2] In a multicenter

[a] Emergency Services, University of Kentucky Chandler Medical Center, 1000 South Limestone Street A.00.403, Lexington, KY 40536, USA; [b] Emergency Services, UK Healthcare, 1000 South Limestone Street A.00.402, Lexington, KY 40536, USA; [c] Emergency Services, University of Kentucky Chandler Medical Center, 1000 South Limestone Street A.00.404, Lexington, KY 40536, USA; [d] Critical Care Services, UK Healthcare Good Samaritan Hospital, 310 South Limestone Street, Lexington, KY 40508, USA
* Corresponding author.
E-mail address: pkhoward@uky.edu

Nurs Clin N Am 49 (2014) 53–60
http://dx.doi.org/10.1016/j.cnur.2013.11.002
0029-6465/14/$ – see front matter © 2014 Elsevier Inc. All rights reserved.

nursing.theclinics.com

study, the researchers illustrated that pain management did not meet patients' expectations for pain relief. These investigators identified a lack of ED research related to pain.[2]

Optimal clinical outcomes are facilitated by adequate pain control. There is support that patients' perceptions of their care, and specifically management of their pain, impacts their clinical outcomes.[3] Patients' perceptions of their illness and functional abilities improved when their pain was reduced. These investigators also suggested that further study may be warranted to examine the relationship between the patient's pain and mental well-being.

Emergency care is episodic, and pain management in the ED may be complicated by long waits, health care professionals' concerns for misuse/abuse, and, more recently, regulatory limitations in some states.[2,4] In 2012, regulations were promulgated in Kentucky that limit the amount of narcotics prescribed in an episodic care setting to a 48-hour supply. This legislation was directed at prescription abuse and "pill mills," yet may have some unintended negative consequences for patients who have limited access to care.[5]

Poor patient satisfaction has been associated with ineffective pain management.[6] A review of qualitative data from patient satisfaction surveys highlighted a poor likelihood to recommend when the patient scored pain control as poor. The voice of the patient showcases how important helpful pain strategies are to perceptions of care.

A limiting factor for effective pain management may be clinical staff attitudes about pain and pain management. An innovative approach to address this was developed from less than desirable patient satisfaction scores directly attributable to pain control. A team of interprofessional stakeholders (ED nursing leadership, ED attending physicians, ED pharmacists, ED registered nurses, pain nurse, ED nursing staff development) was assembled to develop strategies for improvement. It was determined that a multifaceted approach would be used to improve pain management and, indirectly, patient satisfaction scores. The stakeholders' overarching goals were to increase awareness and importance of treating pain by all those who care for ED patients, and reeducate all staff on pain management with an end goal of a comprehensive holistic approach to ED pain management. Pain champions were appointed and included nursing, physician, and pharmacy representation. These interprofessional champions were charged with engaging and educating the staff to improve pain care. Nursing champions attended the "Pain Resource Nurse" (PRN)[7] course to increase their personal knowledge to better educate their peers. Pain champions were critical to the success of the initiative.

An investigation into pain, perceptions, and perceived conflicts of ED staff was developed to gain an understanding about staff-managed pain in an academic medical center. Approval from the medical institutional review board was received for this study; the study objectives can be found in **Box 1**. The study design used a prospective pretest/posttest with a 5-point Likert-type scale that was adapted from the attitudes survey from the PRN course.[7] Letters were sent to emergency nurses and emergency medicine residents requesting voluntary participation in this study. A link to the confidential Internet-based survey was included in the study letter sent via department e-mail (**Table 1**). A review of the baseline survey results revealed areas of knowledge deficit and misperceptions about pain management techniques. Pain champions from the stakeholder team developed "Operation Pain." This project was developed to promote effective pain measures for every patient every time. There were several educational aspects of Operation Pain: brief themed pain management techniques during the preshift huddles for a week (**Box 2**), a banner in the ED, and language on the white board in each patient room "tell us if you have pain." The pain

Box 1
Study objectives
Determine the impact of education on ED staff perception related to pain management.
Describe 2 methods to measure staff knowledge of pain management.
Investigate effects of pain management education on patient satisfaction scores related to pain.
Determine which pain management strategies are more commonly used by staff.

champions coordinated a 4-hour interprofessional education offering that was mandatory for all clinical staff. Content for the education was modeled from some aspects of the PRN course.[7] Weekly pain pearls were e-mailed to nursing staff by the pain champions who also worked collaboratively with staff development to verify pain management competencies for clinical staff need while leading by example in the clinical arena. After completion of the 4-hour education session and verification of competency, the postsurvey link was sent to staff. The original study protocol was amended to add 6 survey questions about pain management strategies (**Fig. 1**).

DISCUSSION

Seventy-six ED nurses and residents responded to the baseline survey. Thirty-six ED nurses completed the postsurvey. It was unclear why the residents did not complete the postsurvey, although survey fatigue was considered. The mean pretest and

Table 1
Attitudes survey

Attitudes Survey	Strongly Disagree	Disagree	Neutral	Agree	Strongly Agree
Older people can bore you to death talking about pain.	1	2	3	4	5
I like to be known as a person who doesn't complain about pain.	1	2	3	4	5
Older women complain about pain more than older men.	1	2	3	4	5
Men are supposed to be brave and not let anybody know if they have pain.	1	2	3	4	5
Some patients exaggerate their pain as a way of getting attention.	1	2	3	4	5
Patients are often embarrassed to tell their nurse that they're hurting.	1	2	3	4	5
Learning to live with pain builds character.	1	2	3	4	5
Life is painful. There is no getting around that.	1	2	3	4	5
By suffering pain in this life, we are purifying ourselves for life to come.	1	2	3	4	5
If patients can still get around or do things, I have to wonder if they are in that much pain.	1	2	3	4	5

Box 2
Operation pain

Daily Huddle Focus:

Monday: ABCs of Pain Assessment

- A – ask regularly
- B – believe patient's report of pain
- C – choose treatment options based on assessment
- D – deliver interventions in a timely way
- E – evaluate treatment effectiveness by reassessment

Tuesday: Set a Realistic Pain Goal

- Achievable
- Mutually acceptable
- Each and every patient

Wednesday: Complete Pain Assessments

- Onset
- Location
- Duration
- Quality
- Intensity
- Type of pain
- Special considerations

Thursday: Use Nonpharmacologic Pain Measures

- 5-minute hand massage
- Distraction
- Heat
- Ice
- Relaxation techniques

Friday: Assess Your Patients' Pain

- Are they getting the right medication
- The right time frame
- The right dose for their type of pain
- Follow-up with your physician

Saturday: Reassess Pain Interventions: Don't Forget to Document What You've Done

- Within 30 minutes of parenteral drug administration
- Within 1 hour of oral medication administration
- With each report of new pain
- With unrelieved pain
- With each report of changes in pain
- Before, during, and after procedures
- Whenever pain is suspected

Sunday: Look for Nonverbal Pain Cues

- Facial expressions
- Verbalizations, vocalizations
- Mental status changes
- Body movements
- Changes in interpersonal interactions
- Changes in activity

posttest scores showed little change for attitudes and were not statistically significant but did trend more positively after the education (**Fig. 2**). Staff reported that they perceived pain differently and had a greater focus on pain interventions after the education. Most significant was the change in patient satisfaction scores related to pain control. Before Operation Pain was implemented, the "how well my pain was managed" mean score was 67.3 (seventh percentile). The quarter following the education and pain champion activities, the "how well my pain was managed" mean score increased to 80.3 (73rd percentile).

Staff responses about pain management strategies were not measured at baseline. The opportunity to learn staff practices regarding pain management (**Fig. 3**) supported a tendency to start with suboptimal management pain control practices, as identified in the Pain and Emergency Medicine Initiative (PEMI) study.[2] Validating these practices led to additional education being provided by the pain champions on the advanced nursing protocols, with more substantive pain management modalities. Advanced nursing protocols are nurse-driven order sets approved by the ED medical

Pain Question			Yes	No
I am an advocate for pain				
I always assess patient's levels on admission				
I routinely re-assess patient's pain after an intervention				
I always assess patient's pain level at/prior to discharge				
I ensure that patient's pain is improved prior to discharge or transfer				
Strategy:	**Distraction**	**Basic Measures ice, elevation**	**NSAIDS**	**Narcotics**
The first pain management technique I use with patients with a pain score less than 4 is:				
The first pain management technique I use with patients with a pain score greater than 4 is:				
The follow-up pain management technique I use with patients with a pain score greater than 4 is:				

Fig. 1. Postsurvey pain management strategies.

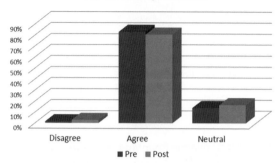

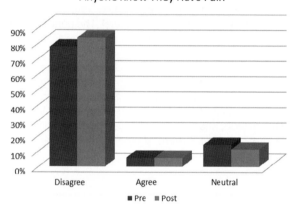

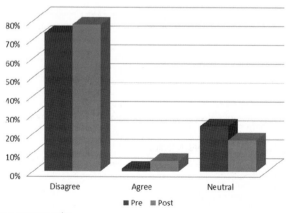

Fig. 2. Attitudes survey results.

The first pain management technique used for pain score <4

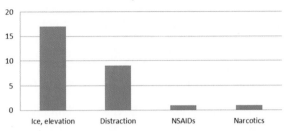

The first pain management technique used for pain >4

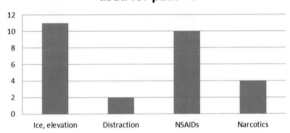

Follow-up pain management techniques for pain score >4

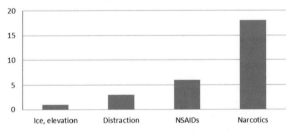

Fig. 3. Pain management survey results.

staff. The nurse can choose to implement these protocols based on clinical assessment. This is most effective when the ED is crowded, delays are likely, and the patient is experiencing moderate to severe pain.

The strengths associated with this study were a potential Hawthorne effect and a meaningful change in patients' pain control as measured in the change in patient satisfaction scores. The increased emphasis on effective pain control has resulted in more staff focus on pain management strategies, both nonpharmacologic and pharmacologic measures for all ages. ED clinical staff are committed to ensuring that pain is assessed early, with frequent reassessments postintervention. Limitations of this investigation include disparity between the pretest and posttest sample sizes, as well as lack of homogeneity between the subjects in each sample. These inequities make it difficult to be certain this could be generalized to other EDs.

SUMMARY

According to Saint Augustine, "The greatest evil is physical pain." This is reflected in patients' perceptions of their pain. Pain education and innovative approaches to nurse-driven protocols are essential to ensure the most optimal provision of care and clinical outcomes. ED welcome brochures include information about pain control and the "Universal Pain Tool" in 8 languages. ED staff attitudes have changed over time, and the increased advocacy has benefited their patients. Emergency nurses participating in Operation Pain placed a higher priority on pain management for their patients.

Pain control remains a priority for the ED. Staff perform purposeful rounding to consistently assess pain levels. Pain assessment and interventions are monitored through reports from the electronic medical record on a monthly basis. It is an expectation that 80% of all patients with a pain score greater than 4 will have an intervention completed and documented with reassessment noted. Metrics related to pain interventions are included in the ED dashboard and shared with staff. Patient satisfaction data related to "how well pain was controlled" is disseminated in the weekly note sent to ED nursing and medical staff. Pain is the reason most patients come to the ED, it is nursing's accountability to ensure they receive the appropriate intervention.

REFERENCES

1. Bhuiya F, Pitts S, McCraig L. Emergency department visits for chest pain and abdominal pain: United States, 1999–2008. NCHS Data Brief. Hyattsville (MD): National Center for Health Statistics; 2010. p. 43.
2. Todd K, Ducharme J, Choiniere M, et al. Pain in the emergency department: results of the pain and emergency medicine initiative (PEMI) multicenter study. J Pain 2007;8:460–6.
3. Moss-Morris R, Humphrey K, Johnson M, et al. Patient's perceptions of their pain condition across a multidisciplinary pain management program: do they change and if so does it matter? Clin J Pain 2007;23:558–64.
4. Bergman C. Emergency nurses' perceived barriers to demonstrating caring when managing adult patients' pain. J Emerg Nurs 2012;38:218–25.
5. Commonwealth of Kentucky Legislative Review Commission. KRS Chapter 218A. Available at: http://www.kbml.ky.gov/NR/rdonlyres/DFFF4843-1343-4468-9574-C9BE26CE48CF/0/HouseBill1.pdf. Accessed September 15, 2013.
6. DuPree E, Martin L, Anderson R, et al. Improving patient satisfaction with pain management using six sigma tools. Jt Comm J Qual Patient Saf 2009;35:343–50.
7. Dahl J, Gordon D, Palce J, editors. Pain resource nurse program curriculum and planning guide. Madison (WI): The Resource Center of the Alliance of State Pain Initiatives; 2008.

Reducing Skin Breakdown in Patients Receiving Extracorporeal Membranous Oxygenation

Linda Clements, APRN, CCNS[a],*, Mary Moore, RN, BSN[b],
Thomas Tribble[a], Jill Blake, RN, MSN[a]

KEYWORDS

- Pressure ulcers • Extracorporeal membranous oxygenation
- Critically ill surgical patients • Mechanical circulatory support
- Nurse sensitive indicator

KEY POINTS

- Pressure ulcer prevention is a top priority within nursing practice when it comes to hospital-acquired infections.
- Poor outcomes associated with pressure ulcers include increased length of stay, increased pain and discomfort, decreased patient and family satisfaction, and increased cost.
- Using evidence and clinical experience with the ECMO population, a multidisciplinary team developed three strategies to improve the rate of hospital-acquired pressure ulcers in an ECMO population.

INTRODUCTION

Pressure ulcer prevention is a top priority within nursing practice.[1] The Centers for Medicare and Medicaid Services and the Agency for Healthcare Research and Quality have recognized pressure ulcers as an important metric measuring quality of nursing care and hospital safety.[2] Poor outcomes associated with pressure ulcers include increased length of stay, increased pain and discomfort, decreased patient and family satisfaction, and increased cost.[3] Studies indicate that patients classified as critically ill are at greatest risk for pressure ulcer development.[4,5] Risk factors associated with pressure ulcer development in critical care patients are poor nutritional status, age, altered sensory perception, exposure to moisture, infection, diabetes and severity of illness.[6] In 2009, 3.3% of intensive care unit patients in the United States developed

[a] Nursing Professional Practice, Medical Center, University of Kentucky Chandler, 800 Rose Street, Lexington, KY 40536, USA; [b] Quality and Safety Department, Medical Center, University of Kentucky Chandler, 800 Rose Street, Lexington, KY 40536, USA
* Corresponding author. Medical Center, University of Kentucky Chandler, HA 108, Lexington, KY 40536.
E-mail address: lclem2@email.uky.edu

Nurs Clin N Am 49 (2014) 61–68
http://dx.doi.org/10.1016/j.cnur.2013.11.003   **nursing.theclinics.com**
0029-6465/14/$ – see front matter © 2014 Elsevier Inc. All rights reserved.

a severe facility-acquired pressure ulcer defined as stage III, stage IV, unstageable, or deep tissue injury.[5] Cardiac surgery patients are reported as one of the most at-risk patient populations for developing hospital-acquired pressure ulcers, with incidence rates reported as high as 29.5%.[7] Data on the cost of pressure ulcers vary; however, reported hospitalization treatment costs range from $37,800 to $70,000 with total annual costs in the United States as high as $11 billion.[8]

PRESSURE ULCER DEVELOPMENT IN PATIENTS ON EXTRACORPOREAL MEMBRANOUS OXYGENATION

Through quality monitoring the authors' identified the cardiovascular-thoracic intensive care unit (CVTICU) had a high incidence of pressure ulcers in their patients receiving extracorporeal membranous oxygenation (ECMO) for cardiac and/or pulmonary support. ECMO is a modified form of cardiopulmonary bypass used to provide support to critically ill adults with respiratory or circulatory failure refractory to conventional management strategies.[9] Critically ill patients are defined as those patients who are at high risk for actual or potential life-threatening health problems.[10] There are several factors that make the nursing care for ECMO patients unique as compared to other critically ill intensive care patients. The most important being, patients are wholly dependent on the ECMO circuit for survival. This circumstance demands a level of nursing vigilance and technological expertise greater than required for most other intensive care patients. Many patients on ECMO may require life-saving measures many times during a 12 hour shift.[11] Adult ECMO treatment requires the placement of two large bore catheters (21-23 F). Cannulation for ECMO occurs at the right internal jugular vein, right common femoral vein, femoral artery, or chest. Bleeding is the most common complication of ECMO, largely due to the requirement of systematic anticoagulation. Therefore, bleeding and decannulation of the ECMO catheter are of great concern when mobilizing the patient. Blood flow, while on ECMO, is directed to the brain and the heart, organs that are most responsive to increased perfusion pressure and least dependent on arteriolar tone. At the same time, blood flow is decreased to organs in which vasculature is the least sensitive to increased perfusion pressure, like the skin and skeletal muscle.[11] Peripheral tissue perfusion during ECMO can become constricted, despite seemingly adequate central hemodynamics and oxygenation. The adequate central hemodynamics and oxygenation can lead the nurse to believe that skin tissue perfusion is adequate, when it actually may be at risk for pressure ulcer development.[11] In 2010, our unit admitted approximately one ECMO patient per month. However, in 2012, the number of ECMO patients admitted to our unit tripled at three per month. In 2012, it came to our attention through a patient safety report that one of our patients on ECMO had developed a deep tissue injury. A retrospective chart review of ECMO patients revealed a pressure ulcer rate of 41% in 2010 and 65% in 2011. Safety concerns related to hemodynamic instability, poor perfusion and dislodgement or accidental decannulation of the ECMO catheter were verbalized by nursing staff as possible reasons contributing to the lack of repositioning ECMO patients thus increasing the risk of pressure ulcers in this population.[12]

OUR UNIT/DEVELOPING A MULTIDISCIPLINARY TEAM

In January of 2012, a multidisciplinary group comprised of CTVICU bedside nurses, physicians, the clinical nurse specialist and the wound care specialist began developing a focused and aggressive plan to reduce the rate of hospital-acquired pressure ulcers in our ECMO patient population. Our CTVICU is a 16-bed unit. The unit patient population includes those who have received cardiac surgery, heart or lung transplants or mechanical circulatory support devices. The nursing staff consists of more than 70 nurses with approximately 10 nurses for each shift of 16 patients. The unit is staffed with approximately two to three nursing care technicians per shift. The goals of this multidisciplinary group are found in **Box 1**.

LITERATURE REVIEW

A targeted search of the available literature was conducted to identify clinical evidence on risk factors related to pressure ulcer development in critically ill ECMO patients. This was a purposeful search to identify the best quality clinical studies and review articles rather than a systematic literature search. The papers identified were reviewed for relevance, with the key points from pertinent studies highlighted. The literature was very limited related to the nursing care of ECMO patients. Several studies were found reporting the risk for developing a pressure ulcer in the critically ill intensive care patient. Evidence reports prolonged pressure concentrated over bony prominences is thought to be the single most important factor in pressure ulcer formation.[13] Prolonged high pressure results in local tissue ischemia, which is associated with local perfusion failure of capillaries which leads to tissue necrosis.[13] Risk factors that predispose critically ill patients to pressure ulcer development are prolonged immobility (physiologically intolerant to turning, nurses fear of injury to patient during turning), poor nutrition, older age, poor local skin perfusion, vasopressor infusions, decreased sensation and time on operating (OR) table.[14–16] The multidisciplinary team decided to focus on risk factors that were the most relevant to their ECMO population. These were prolonged mobility (poor physiologic tolerance to turning), fear of patient injury during turning, time spent on the operating table and the infusion of vasopressors.

Poor Physiologic Tolerance to Turning and Fear of Patient Injury During Turning

Prolonged immobility can cause patient's to have a physiological intolerance to turning.[14] Cardiovascular changes in heart rate, stroke volume and cardiac output have been reported with manual turning.[14,15] Normally, the body adjusts for position changes, however with prolonged immobility, protective mechanisms such as vestibular and baroreceptor responses are disrupted.[16,17] This disruption can be caused by decreased stroke volume resulting in a reduced baroreceptor reflex and neurohomonal effects on plasma volume.[16,17] If the turn is tolerated, the patient should recover and return to their baseline cardiovascular parameters in 5-10 minutes.[18] Several practices are recommended in the literature that could improve the critical care patient's intolerance to repositioning making turning easier. These include continuous lateral rotation therapy, which is delivered by continuous motion equipped bed frames and "off-loading".[19–24] Patients who are physiologically intolerant to a full lateral turn may benefit from continuous lateral rotation therapy(CLRT).[20] It has been suggested that CLRT may be able to retrain patients to tolerate turning because the speed of

---

Box 1
Goals

- Identify risk factors associated with the development of pressure ulcers in our patients on ECMO.
- Develop effective strategies to prevent pressure ulcers in patients on ECMO.
- Develop methods to monitor for hospital-acquired pressure ulcer development in our ECMO population.

the turn is slower than a manual turn, allowing more time for equilibration of plasma volume.[22] Another mechanism to prevent pressure ulcers in patients who are intolerant to manual turning is to institute slight, subtle and frequent position changes, through "off-loading".[23,24] Off-loading has been defined as any measure to eliminate abnormal pressure points to promote healing or to prevent pressure ulcers.[23] Off-loading is more effective when the pressure is dispersed evenly over a wide area. Pillows, special padded boots and turning wedges are often used as off-loading devices in the bedridden patient.[24] Surgical site bleeding and hemorrhage are major complications for ECMO patients related to their need for systemic heparinzation and the placement of two large bore catheters for ECMO treatment. The dislodgement of these catheters would place the ECMO patient at high risk for blood loss. The fear of the dislodgement of patient tubes and catheters during positioning is a major concern of critical care nurses and can be a deterrent to turning critically ill patients.[25] In one study, researchers found that 34% of bedside nurses worry about the dislodgement of tubes and potential injury to patients during turning.[21] It is suggested that repositioning be planned and adequate resources (respiratory therapists, perfusionist, extra nurses to hold tubes and drains) be available at the bedside to prevent tubes and catheters from dislodging during turning.[25]

Time on Operating Table and Intravenous Infusion of Vasoactive Drips

As high as 23% of hospital acquired pressure ulcers have been shown to have originated in the operating room.[26] It is often thought that time on the operating table is insufficient to generate a pressure ulcer. Research shows that pressure ulcers can develop in as little as 1-4 hours depending on the patient and their severity of illness.[26] During surgical procedures, patients are immobile, unable to change their position and also unable to feel pain related to anesthesia.[27] In our institution, durations of cardiac surgeries can range from 3 hours to 10 hours depending on the reason for the surgery. Several articles found time on the operating table to contribute to pressure ulcer development in intensive care patients.[27,28] For example, in a sample of 125 patients undergoing various surgical procedures, researchers found older age, time on the operating room table, diastolic episodes of hypotension, preoperative Braden scores, serum albumin levels, and total protein levels to be moderately predictive of developing a pressure ulcer postsurgery.[28] One model using time on the operating table, extracorporeal circulation, and age emerged as the best predictor of pressure ulcer development in surgical patients in this study.[28] The National Pressure advisory panel suggests the use of pressure redistributing surface, proper positioning, elevation of heels during surgery and to initially reposition patients in the post-operative period different than they were positioned during surgery to prevent pressure ulcers in the operating room.[29]

Critical care patients often require pharmacological support such as vasopressors for their blood pressure. Commonly used vasopressors are epinephrine, norepinephrine, vasopressin, phenylephrine and dopamine. These drugs are potent vasoconstrictors that elevate the blood pressure by shunting blood away from the perphery to the vital organs. This action, though much needed to preserve vital organ function, deprives the capillary beds of much needed oxygen and nutrients.[30] Recommendations to prevent pressure ulcers in patients on vasopressor infusions are to closely monitor skin for signs of decreased tissue perfusion while the patient is on the infusion.[31] Using the evidence and clinical experience with the ECMO population, the multidisciplinary team developed three strategies to improve the rate of hospital-acquired pressure ulcers. These included increasing staff awareness of pressure ulcer risk factors in

ECMO patients, developing a turning guideline and a skin bundle and the use of clinical coaching at the bedside to educate and train nurses in pressure ulcer prevention.

STRATEGY #1: INCREASE STAFF AWARENESS OF PRESSURE ULCER RISK FACTORS IN ECMO PATIENTS

Formal mandatory education sessions on pressure ulcer prevention were planned and implemented by the CNS. Nurses were given patient scenarios to enhance for discussion and critical thinking about pressure ulcer prevention. This technique engaged nurses in planning and anticipating skin care needs for our ECMO patients. Root cause analyses were completed by the clinical nurse specialist and the bedside nurses on all patients who developed a pressure ulcer (any stage) in the unit. During the root cause analysis, nurses were given sections of the chart to review. Each section represented a factor placing a patient at increased risk for developing a pressue ulcer. (i.e. vasopressor infusions, documented turned every two hours, mean arterial pressure >65). Documentation was inconsistent at times on patient turning and skin care compliance. If patients were documented they were "too unstable to be turned", nurses were asked to suggest other alternatives for relieving skin pressure and preventing breakdown. Staff were asked to perform at least three skin care documentation audits per month. The documentation audits in our unit have been key to improving the rate of hospital-acquired pressure ulcers in this population. Audit and feedback has been used for years to change nursing clinical practice behavior. In a Cochrane review, audit with feedback was found to be an effective strategy to change practice especially when adherence with baseline practice is low.[30] The monthly skin audit were completed for three months with compliance improving steadily.

STRATEGY #2: DEVELOPMENT OF A TURNING GUIDELINE AND SKIN CARE BUNDLE

Using the literature review and clinical experience as a guide, a protocol was developed for turning hemodynamically unstable patients. The protocol included parameters that deem the patient hemodynamically unstable, recommended evidence-based interventions for turning the unstable patients, and a guideline for using continious lateral rotation. A "skin bundle" was created to be used for patients at the time of ECMO initiation. The skin bundle included the use of a speciality bed if needed, an automatic wound and ostomy nurse consult and a special "gel positioner". This gel positioner (Z-flo Sundance Enterprise inc. New York) was trialed and found to be very helpful in "offloading" critically ill patients who had poor physiological tolerance to turning. This protocol and the skin bundle assisted nurses to integrate new knowledge and decision-making skills concerning pressure ulcer prevention into their practice.

STRATEGY #3: USE OF COACHING TO PROMOTE PRESSURE ULCER PREVENTION

Many approaches have been used to promote the adoption of evidence-based research into practice. Several studies have shown that clinical coaching is an effective strategy for assisting in the development of nursing practice in order to positively affect patient outcomes.[31,32] Clinical coaching is defined as the promotion of skills for using processes such as critical thinking and problem solving.[31] Coaching is focused tool that uses conversations at the bedside to infuse evidence-based research into practice.[31] Educational sessions concerning the promotion of skin integrity and the recognition of early pressure ulcer development were offered to staff. Daily skin rounds were initiated and included visualization of the patient's skin (by the clinical nurse specialist and the bedside nurse), bedside instruction on

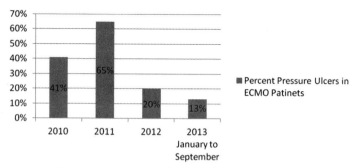

Fig. 1. Percentage of pressure ulcers in patients on ECMO.

interventions to promote healthy skin and instruction on offloading pressure points. During episodes of bedside coaching, family members were often involved in discussions about their role in pressure ulcer prevention. Skin rounds were performed daily for three months. Then as nurses began becoming more proficient at recognizing breaches in skin integrity and applying appropriate skin management techniques, skin rounds were moved out to weekly, where they remain. Clinical coaching at the bedside provided real time expert "feedback" to the bedside nurse. Providing real-time feedback to nurses concerning patient care situations provides objective data about the nurses' performance and allows bedside nurses time to engage in intellectual discussion and self-reflection on their behavior.[33] Nurses were encouraged to use peer-to-peer consultation for any skin questions when the CNS was not available.

SUMMARY

The multidisciplinary team developed a plan for monitoring pressure ulcer development in our ECMO population. The nurses were to use the patient safety network system to report any breach in skin integrity. A monthly meeting is in place to discuss the frequency of pressure ulcers in our unit and to institute any changes that were needed. The CNS receives a daily list of patients with pressure ulcers noting their stage and location. During the next 12 months, in 2012, the pressure ulcer rate in our ECMO patients decreased by 44%. So far in the year 2013, the pressure ulcer rate in our ECMO patients is 13% (see **Fig. 1**).

This program emphasizes the value of using evidence-based approaches to improve practice. This multifaceted approach to a change in practice seems to have resulted in a significant change in nursing culture concerning protecting critically ill ECMO patients from the development of pressure ulcers. This was a successful project and the work continues. We have learned through constant evaluation of our processes and continual focus on patient safety issues that most pressure ulcers can be avoided.

REFERENCES

1. Fact sheet. Serious Adverse Events Working Group. Available at: http://www.qualityforum.org. Accessed March 19, 2008.
2. AHRQ's National Guideline Clearinghouse Guideline Synthesis on Pressure Ulcers. Prevention of pressure ulcers. Available at: http://www.guideline.gov/syntheses/synthesis.aspx?id?25078. Accessed July 23, 2013.

3. Berlowitz D, VanDeusen LC, Parker V, et al. Preventing pressure ulcers in hospitals. A toolkit for improving quality of care. Rockville (MD): Agency for Healthcare Research and Quality; 2011. Available at: http://www.ahrq.gov/research/ltc/pressureulcertoolkit/. Accessed July 24, 2013.

4. de Laat EH, Schoonhoven L, Pickers P, et al. Epidemiology, risk and prevention of pressure ulcers in critically ill patients: a literature review. J Wound Care 2006;16: 269–75.

5. VanGilder C, Amlung S, Harrison P, et al. Results of the 2008–2009 International Pressure Ulcer Prevalence TM Survey and a 3-year, acute care, unit-specific analysis. Ostomy Wound Manage 2009;55(11):39–45.

6. Shahain ES, Dassen T, Halfens RJ. Pressure ulcer prevalence in intensive care patients: a cross sectional study. J Eval Clin Prac 2008;14(4):563–8.

7. Feuchtinger J, Halfens RJ, Dassen T. Pressure ulcer risk factors in cardiac surgery: a review of the research literature. Heart Lung 2005;34(6):375–85.

8. Russo CA, Steiner C, Spector W. Hospitalizations related to pressure ulcers among adults 18 years and older, 2006. HCUP Statistical Brief 64. Rockville (MD): Agency for Healthcare Research and Quality; 2008. Available at: http://www.hcupus.ahrq.gov/reports/statbriefs/sb64.pdf. Accessed January 10, 2013.

9. Massetti M, Tasle M, Le Page O, et al. Back from irreversibility: extracorporeal life support for prolonged cardiac arrest. Ann Thorac Surg 2005;79:178.

10. Alspach JA. Core Curriculum for Critical Care Nursing. St. Louis (MO): Sanders Elsevier Health Sciences; 2013.

11. Bartlett RH, Roloff DW, Custer JR, et al. Extracorporeal life support: the University of Michigan experience. JAMA 2000;283(7):904–8.

12. Morris PE. Moving our critically ill patients: mobility barriers and benefits. Crit Care Clin 2007;23:1–20.

13. Makhsous M, Priebe M, Bankard J, et al. Measuring tissue perfusion during pressure relief maneuvers: insights into preventing pressure ulcers. The Journal of Spinal Cord Medicine 2007;30(5):497–507.

14. Convertino VA, Doerr DF, Eckberg DL, et al. Head-down bed rest impairs vagal baroreflex responses and provokes orthostatic hypotension. J Appl Physiol (1985) 1990;68:1458–64.

15. Schoonhoven L, Defloor T, van der Tweel I, et al. Risk indicators for pressure ulcers during surgery. Applied Nursing Research 2002;15(3):163–73.

16. Cox J. Pressure ulcer development and vasopressor agents in adult critical care patients: a literature review. Ostomy and Wound Management 2013;59(4):56–60.

17. Winkelman C. Bed rest in health and critical illness: a body systems approach. AACN Adv Crit Care 2009;20(3):254–66.

18. Vollman K. Introduction to progressive mobility. Crit Care Nurse 2010;30:3–5.

19. Winslow EH, Lane LD, Woods RJ. Dangling: a review of relevant physiology, research and practice. Heart Lung 1995;24:263–72.

20. Vollman K. Hemodynamic instability: is it really a barrier to turning critically ill patients? Crit Care Nurse 2012;32:70–5.

21. Winkleman C, Perreboom K. Staff perceived barriers and facilitators. Critical Care Nurse 2010;30:13–6.

22. Washington GT, Macnee CL. Evaluation of outcomes: the effects of continuous lateral rotational therapy. J Nurs Care Qual 2005;20(3):273–82.

23. Armstrong DG, Nguyen HC, Lavery LA, et al. Off-loading the diabetic foot wound: a randomized control trial. Diabetes Care 2001;24(6):1019–22.

24. Wu SC, Jensen JL, Weber AK, et al. Use of pressure offloading devices in diabetic foot ulcers do we practice what we preach? Diabetes Care 2008;31(11):2118–9.

25. Stiller K. Safety issues that should be considered when mobilizing critically ill patients. Critical care clinics 2007;23(1):35–53.
26. Gefen A. How much time does it take to get a pressure ulcer? Integrated evidence from human, animal and in vitro studies. Ostomy Wound Manage 2008; 54:26–35.
27. Papantonio CT, Wallop KB, Kolodner KB. Sacral ulcers following cardiac surgery: incidence and risks. Adv Wound Care 1994;7:24–6.
28. Kemp MG, Keithley JK, Morreale B, et al. Factors that contribute to pressure sores in surgical patients. Res Nurs Health 1990;13:293–301.
29. European Pressure Ulcer Advisory Panel and National Pressure Ulcer Advisory Panel. Treatment of pressure ulcers: quick reference guide. Washington, DC: National Pressure Ulcer Advisory Panel; 2009.
30. Jamtvedt G, Young JM, Kristoffersen DT, et al. Audit and feedback: effects on professional practice and health care outcomes. Cochrane Database Syst Rev 2006;(2):CD000259.
31. Gordon SJ, Melillo KD, Nannini A, et al. Bedside coaching to improve nurses' recognition of delirium. The Journal of Neuroscience Nursing 2013;45(5):288–93.
32. Ervin N. Clinical coaching: a strategy for enhancing evidence-based nursing practice. Clin Nurse Spec 2005;19(6):296–301.
33. Grealish L. The skills of coach are an essential element in clinical learning. The Journal of Nursing Education 2000;39(5):231.

Engaging the Learner by Bridging the Gap Between Theory and Clinical Competence

The Impact of Concept Mapping and Simulation as Innovative Strategies for Nurse-Sensitive Outcome Indicators

Therese Jamison, DNP, ACNP-BC*, Gail A. Lis, DNP, ACNP-BC

KEYWORDS

- Nurse-sensitive indicators • Clinical competency • Meaningful learning • Simulation
- Concept mapping

KEY POINTS

- Nurse-sensitive indicators have been determined to be an integral part of quality initiatives; these performance measures are a means to highlight competency in relation to nursing care.
- The strength of combining the 2 learning strategies of concept mapping and simulation provides theoretical support for enhancing the construction and assimilation of knowledge related to nurse-sensitive indicators as a means to develop meaningful learning.
- A concept map is a visual representation of knowledge with pathways that connect ideas in ways that make sense to the learner.
- Simulation provides translation of theory knowledge into practice and has the potential to augment cognitive thinking and ultimately problem-solving, thus supporting clinical competence.

INTRODUCTION

The American Nurses Association[1] contends that the public has a right to expect competence from professional nurses, and the profession has a responsibility to guide and develop this competency.[1] Ultimately, the main purpose for ensuring competence is for public protection. The protection of the public is in direct alignment with the call

No conflict of interest or disclosures for T. Jamison or G. Lis.

College of Nursing and Health, Madonna University, 36600 Schoolcraft, Livonia, MI 48150, USA

* Corresponding author.

E-mail address: tjamison@madonna.edu

by the Institute of Medicine[2,3] for quality and safety in the health care system. Nurse-sensitive indicators have been determined to be an integral part of quality initiatives; these performance measures are a means to highlight competency in relation to nursing care.[4]

Quality and safety in the health care system depend on the complex interactions of competent individuals and competent systems. Developing and understanding this complexity must begin in the academic setting and continue on in the professional workplace. Quality, in itself, is not a simple construct. Quality is a complex process that is difficult to take apart. If nurses view quality as a simple entity or task, then they are not likely to understand all of the pieces that impact a particular quality measure. The quality measure becomes viewed as a task instead of a process. Nurse-sensitive indicators are the claim of nursing as a profession.[4] To make this happen, emerging nurses and practicing nurses must learn and appreciate the importance of nursing outcomes and how their contributions can offer a claim to the profession. Understanding the implications of nursing outcomes and developing ownership of the process must begin in the early onset of professional nursing education and carry through into the practice environment. The purpose of this article is to appreciate innovative education strategies to understand and develop best practice as related to nurse-sensitive indicators.

NURSE-SENSITIVE INDICATORS/CLINICAL COMPETENCY

As indicated, nurse-sensitive indicators are determined to be the best-quality benchmark to evaluate nursing practice. Nurse-sensitive indicator or nursing-performance outcomes are defined as "those that are relevant, based on nurses' scope and domain of practice and for which there are empirical evidence linking nursing inputs and interventions to the outcomes."[5] The National Quality Forum delineates nurse-sensitive indicators as not only an outcome, but also a process as well, that is impacted by many factors.[6] The idea of process implies that there may be several variables that need to be considered in order for a particular outcome to occur. An outcome is not achieved in isolation. If an outcome measure is viewed as simply a task that needs to be accomplished, versus a process that impacts an outcome, there is likely to be little "buy in" from the staff to recognize the importance of achieving a particular outcome, and even more concerning, not achieving the outcome at all. If outcomes are not achieved to a satisfactory level, then it is likely that the nursing care could be considered less than satisfactory or even incompetent. Furthermore, if outcome achievement is equated with quality, and quality is equated with competence, ultimately, nurse-sensitive indicators can be conceptualized as a direct reflection of clinical competence.

Although clinical competency is difficult to define, ideas intrinsic to understanding clinical competency include clinical depth and breadth of knowledge, critical thinking and analytic skills, clinical inquiry, synthesis of data, clinical judgment, and clinical decision-making.[7] The attributes associated with clinical competence reflect higher cognitive processes. Lasater[8] supports the idea that nurses will require a higher level of knowledge to enter the work force.

Finkleman and Kenner[9] denote that critical thinking, clinical reasoning, and clinical judgment are important to effective nursing practice. Critical thinking enables nurses to create and examine questions and problems, use intuition, clarify and evaluate evidence, and become a change agent.[9] Critical thinking allows the nurse to question a particular outcome, use experience to offer suggestions on how improvements might occur, and review the evidence for "fit" to a particular patient situation. It is imperative for the nurse to remember that not all evidence will fit every patient. Critical thinking supports open-mindedness and seeks solutions that might be outside the norm.[10] Clinical judgment requires more than recall and understanding of content; it is more than identifying a nurse-sensitive indicator has been met. Clinical judgment allows the nurse to understand the performance measure, analyze the process, and determine how it can be improved.[9]

MEANINGFUL LEARNING

The challenge for educators is to develop and stimulate higher cognitive processes and in essence enhance meaningful learning, which is true for academic education as well as for staff development. Meaningful learning is the result of cognitive, affective, and psychomotor domains of learning and evolves from cognitive learning theory.[11] Cognitive learning is an active process that involves a variety of perspectives that according to Braungart and coworkers[12] determines how a person perceives, interprets, and reorganizes the information into something that makes sense to them. As this occurs, each person's cognitive structure is developed. Therefore, learning is different for everyone because perception, interpretation, and reorganization are likely to vary among individuals. The primary emphasis of cognitive learning theory is the understanding and attainment of knowledge and not simply how to acquire a new behavior or perform a particular task.[12] Furthermore, cognitive theories seek to explain complex learning and support the meaning of the situation versus a specific behavior.[10]

A key idea to meaningful learning is that it is different for everyone. Construction of knowledge is learner-centered and dynamic in nature. Constructivist education is based on 4 hypotheses: (1) knowledge depends on past construction—integration of what is known and what is new promotes learning; (2) constructions are developed through assimilation of new knowledge into a preexisting cognitive structure; (3) learners must be able to construct their own knowledge—each individual has their own cognitive structure that has developed over time as a result of exposure to different learning situations; (4) meaningful learning occurs through reflection and "scaffolding" of new knowledge—assimilation of new knowledge into a preexisting cognitive structure occurs to form a more highly differentiated cognitive structure.[13]

Transformation of knowledge occurs when learning becomes meaningful. This transformation does not occur unless it can be related to something that is tangible, and this is often difficult to do.[14] In the health care setting, professional registered nurses are faced with quality care issues that determine patient outcomes. Performance measures or indicators are impacted by multiple variables and are typically a moving target. In order for these performance measures to be meaningful, the professional registered nurse must be able to appreciate the complexity of the variables and construct meaning out of what is experienced from what is already known; in essence, new knowledge is constructed, or taken in, and assimilated into, to create a scaffold upon preexisting knowledge. Once a learner recognizes the importance of constructing new knowledge from existing knowledge, the process of learning becomes a challenge to embrace instead of a burden to bear.

Meaningful learning has the potential to develop the necessary skills for complex problem-solving and development of competence that is called for by the leading nursing organizations.[15] Problem-solving is a key competence that incorporates clinical judgment and reasoning and an outcome that results from the process of critical thinking. The use of active learning strategies that develop meaningful learning is necessary to support the professional registered nurse in constructing knowledge related to nurse-sensitive outcomes and the relationship to quality care. If nurse-sensitive indicators are to be "the claim to the profession," then undergraduate and graduate nursing curricula as well as the professional workplace should provide learning opportunities that enhance this essential competency. The nurse-sensitive indicators are likely to change over time and will be impacted by a variety of patient situations and institutional and societal circumstances.

It is imperative that the clinical nurse have a voice in identifying priorities and determining select nurse-sensitive indicators by which nursing care is evaluated. With this voice, there will be an appreciation of the complexity of the process that involves evaluation of the structure, process, and overall outcome of a select indicator, creating a perfect opportunity to provide the emerging nurse with foundational concepts, the practicing nurse with additional knowledge to scaffold on top of what is already learned, and to evaluate how evidence is translated into practice. It could provide the graduate nurse further assimilate assessment data to translate current evidence into practice and/or develop new evidence to support the science of nursing.

The cycle should be endless. In order for this to happen, learning strategies need to be incorporated that will sustain the cycle. Concept mapping and simulation are 2 active learning strategies that have been used among educators. Both strategies have been used by nurse educators in isolation but not in combination. The strength of combining the 2 learning strategies of concept mapping and simulation provide theoretical support for enhancing the construction and assimilation of knowledge related to nurse-sensitive indicators as a means to develop meaningful learning. The use of these learning strategies is applicable to both academic and health care settings.

CONCEPT MAPPING

From a conceptual standpoint, concept maps are defined as "declarative models of personal understanding comprising concept labels to identify specific ideas and explanatory links that give these ideas meaning."[16(pp222)] Concepts are ideas that represent knowledge and a map is a guide that determines a particular pathway. A concept map, therefore, is a visual representation of knowledge with pathways that connect ideas in ways that make sense to the learner.[17]

Concept maps are constructed from concepts and linking words that are arranged in some type of hierarchical order that typically trends from broad to specific. The concepts are isolated by a geometric structure that is connected to another concept by a line depicted with a directional arrow. This connection is referred to as a proposition. A linking word between concepts provides a brief explanation of the relationship. Cross-links provide the connection among multiple concepts to demonstrate synthesis of concepts; this reflects higher order thinking.[17]

In order for nurses to understand the importance of nurse-sensitive indicators to the profession of nursing, they must be able to appreciate what a nurse-sensitive indicator is, the variables that could impact a particular outcome, and how this outcome will impact the care they provide. Understanding the concept of nurse-sensitive indicators will come from foundational knowledge provided in the academic and staff development setting. The variables that impact a particular outcome can be sorted out by examining both the structure and the process. Duffy[18] points out that patient outcomes are multifaceted and are impacted by the setting, patient-specific factors, and interpersonal aspects of care. The structure might include staff-ratio, inter- and intraprofessional relationships, and available support staff. The process might include familiarity with evidence-based guidelines used to support the indicator, ease with which guidelines can be implemented, and perhaps barriers to implementation.

A concept map is an active learning strategy that allows a learner to organize their thinking and highlight variables thought to impact a particular outcome; this could be done through linkages among the structure, process, and outcome concepts. The linkages will provide insight as the learner may realize that there is something in the structure that impacts the process, which ultimately impacts the outcome; or there is something in the process that might impact the structure, which ultimately impacts the outcome. The learning becomes meaningful because the learner is able to assimilate new knowledge from the variables that are outlined within the concepts. That insight occurs because of assimilation that takes place within a learner's cognitive structure. The learner is using skills associated with critical thinking that is important to clinical judgment. Del Bueno[19] purports that clinical judgment requires more than recall: it necessitates the ability to analyze and synthesize knowledge.

The use of concept maps to understand nurse-sensitive indicators can be used in undergraduate and graduate education as well as in staff development. A concept map developed by an undergraduate student might have simple hierarchical structure with single linkages between structure, process, and outcome. The undergraduate student would recognize that evidence exists that supports a particular indicator. It would be expected that the graduate student concept map be more complex that identifies cross-links among concepts. The graduate student would integrate the evidence within the concepts to demonstrate translation into practice. The staff nurse concept map could be developed over time as part of a unit project. The concept map could be a poster board displayed in the conference room that reflects input from all members of the health care team associated with a particular unit. Inter- and intraprofessional collaboration would be encouraged as inputs to the concept map could be color-coded to reflect a particular care provider group. Additional learning may occur as each person contributes to the concept map and reflects on what others have to offer (**Figs. 1** and **2**).

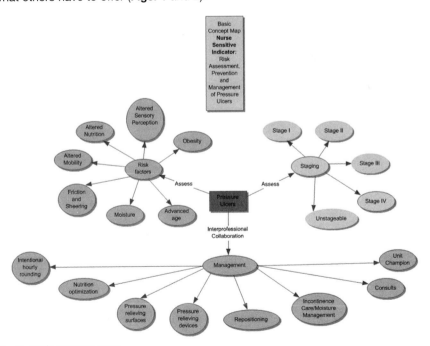

Fig. 1. Basic concept map.

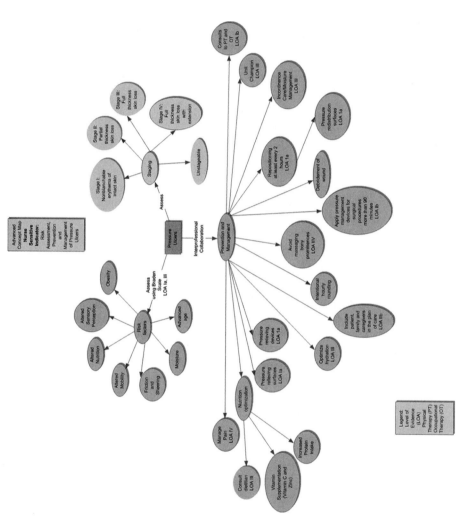

Fig. 2. Advanced concept map.

SIMULATION

Simulation, like concept mapping, is an active learning strategy that supports meaningful learning through constructivism. Simulation provides the opportunity for learners to construct their own learning as they experience new situations.[10] Learning will be different for each individual because the learning that is constructed will be based on different knowledge that is brought to the experience. The new experience will be integrated with the old experience to create new meaning. The interactive learning environment that simulation provides allows the learner to develop links between and among concepts.[20] The connections made between and among concepts in simulation provide the experiential understanding that also helps to solidify learning.

Unlike concept mapping, simulation provides the opportunity for the learner to physically manipulate the experience, provides translation of theory knowledge into practice, and has the potential to augment cognitive thinking and ultimately problem-solving.

Simulation supports clinical competence. "Nursing competence involves the acquisition of relevant knowledge, the development of psychomotor skills, and the ability to apply the knowledge and skills appropriately in a given context."[21(pp74)]

COMBINING THE EDUCATION STRATEGIES

The combination of concept mapping and simulation provides a sound theoretical foundation to support meaningful learning for nurse-sensitive indicators. The 2 active learning strategies support the underlying context of Kolb's experiential learning theory. Kolb[22] posits that "learning is the process whereby knowledge is created through the transformation of experience" (p 38). Kolb's theory is cyclical and is composed of 4 stages; the learner may enter the cycle at any point but must complete all 4 stages in order for knowledge to be created.[23]

The concept map will provide a guide for conceptual learning that the learner can use to prepare for the simulation (forming abstract concepts, testing in new situations). The simulation will provide the experiential contact that will assist the learner to assimilate further what is in place on the concept map to what they have physically experienced. The learner may use an element from an evidence-based guideline that is identified on the concept map to guide the assessment during the simulation or determine an appropriate intervention based on level of evidence (concrete experience). The debriefing process that occurs after simulation allows the learner to reflect on the process and determine how their particular actions impact patient care (reflective observation). This process could continue again in the clinical setting as nurse-sensitive indicators are conceptualized, implemented, and then evaluated. **Fig. 3** portrays the integration of concept mapping into Kolb's cycle of experiential learning. The process to follow describes the application of concept mapping and simulation across undergraduate and graduate curricula and staff development as a vehicle to translate nurse-sensitive indicators to meaningful nursing practice.

THE PROCESS OF USING CONCEPT MAPPING AND SIMULATION IN GRADUATE EDUCATION

The authors have formulated a model of using both concept mapping and simulation to enhance the education of Adult-Gerontology Acute Care Nurse Practitioner students in a Midwestern University setting. The process includes the presentation of concepts related to a particular topic along with objectives and evidence-based

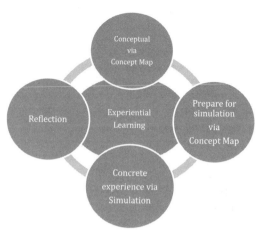

Fig. 3. Integration of concept mapping into Kolb's cycle of experiential learning.

practice guidelines. The faculty posts this information in an on-line format (blackboard) a week before the faculty presenting in a didactic face-to-face environment with the students. During this face-to-face time, the students are encouraged to participate in class discussions related to the topic as well as to case studies. The students are then randomly assigned to a group of 3 to formulate a concept map based on a case scenario as related to the concepts presented in the didactic sessions. A group of 3 students has been used to enhance experiential learning. Larger groups of students typically do not allow for an intensive learning experience. Students are provided with instructions on how to develop a concept map with exemplar examples provided. Potential computerized programs for concept map development (eg, cmap and Inspiration) are provided to the student groups. Hand-drawn concept maps are also accepted by faculty. In essence, the concept map includes the vital information pertaining to the case study, potential changes in the patient's assessment, the development of the differential diagnoses, as well as the clinical practice guidelines and level of evidence as discussed in the literature. These guidelines should not be applied in a "cookbook" fashion, but used as a tool to assist in decision-making for individualized care. Examples of case studies used with this aggregate of students include a patient with a nosocomial urinary tract infection, a patient with a history of atrial fibrillation who is admitted with an ST segment myocardial infarction, as well as a patient with exacerbation of chronic obstructive pulmonary disease.

The nurse practitioner (NP) students come to the simulation with their concept map at an assigned time. They are expected to come in clinical attire (scrubs and a laboratory coat) with necessary equipment (stethoscope, concept map, downloaded programs for reference to medication dosages, and so on). Professional attire promotes a "real" practice environment for the students. The NP students are randomly assigned to 1 of 3 roles, 2 NPs and a staff nurse. A high-fidelity simulator is used in the simulation laboratory rooms that are hard-wired with communication devices. The simulation room mimics the clinical environment with a patient bed, wall unit with oxygen and suction, simulator manikin, beside table, sink, and monitor system. Equipment is stored in a crash cart with medications, intravenous fluids, as well as other equipment that may be anticipated being used during the simulation exercise. The simulation laboratory coordinator provides the students with a presimulation briefing on the process of the simulation to include the capabilities of the high-fidelity simulator, how laboratory tests and other diagnostics are ordered and then provided to the students via the simulator's monitor screen, and where equipment is located and encourages the students to write on a "white board" as the simulation progresses. The "white board" is used to record the initial assessment, laboratory and diagnostics results, interventions ordered and instituted, as well as the change in the simulator's response.

The NP faculty, along with the simulation laboratory coordinator, has programmed the simulator to respond to the NP student's interventions. In the authors' university setting, the faculty is located in another room and views the students via a one-way glass window. The faculty can respond to the student's questions of the patient using a headset. If the students formulate an appropriate assessment of the patient and differential diagnosis as well as institute the evidence-based practice guidelines, the simulator's clinical condition improves; in contrast, if the students do not follow the guidelines, the simulator's clinical condition declines. For example, the patient with the nosocomial urinary tract infection can progress to septic shock; the patient with atrial fibrillation and ST segment myocardial infarction can decline to acute decompensated heart failure with resultant cardiogenic shock, and in the patient with exacerbation of chronic obstructive pulmonary disease, a decline may be seen to require intubation and mechanical ventilation. The time with the simulator is typically 30 minutes.

After the simulation activity, the NP students and faculty proceed to a conference room for debriefing. It is here where the students are encouraged to reflect on best practice, pearls, and pitfalls of their simulation. What the student group did well or could have aligned better with the clinical practice guidelines is discussed. Questions for the students can also include the affective domain for learning, for example, "How did this simulation activity make you feel?" Faculty provides feedback on their teamwork, communication, decision-making, and the simulation patient outcomes. The students then write an after-simulation reflection as it relates to the Adult-Gerontology Acute Care Nurse Practitioner competencies from the American Association of Colleges of Nursing.[23] Students are encouraged to select 3 to 5 competencies and relate these competencies back to the simulation activity. Individual as well as group participation is graded on the simulation activity (**Table 1**). The last piece to this process is an

Table 1
Grading rubric for concept mapping and simulation experience

Criteria	Possible Points	Comments/Earned Points
Completion of concept map that reflects integration of group thinking	30	
Documentation of appropriate clinical practice guidelines with identified level of evidence; integrated into concept maps	10	
Assessment and diagnostics (verbalizes changes in clinical status, diagnostic tests with rationale) Verbalizes differential diagnosis	20	
Implementation of clinical practice guidelines (focus on evidence, safety, and quality)	20	
Individual participation	10	
Postreflection: integration of adult gerontology acute care NP competencies with specific examples from simulation	10	

on-line examination that covers the concepts of the simulation. The examination is typically 25 questions, timed for 1 hour.

Although formal quantitative data for on-line examination achievement are forthcoming, the faculty author's observation is that students perform very well on the on-line examinations. Students relate that the process of faculty-led didactic presentation, student group concept map development, simulation activity, and debriefing offers them an enhanced opportunity to embrace evidence-based practice guidelines as well as to perform on the on-line examinations. The students comments included: "This simulation was extremely educational because it revealed my need to trust my gut"; "Because I forgot this assessment during simulation, I am much more likely to remember this in practice"; "Each simulation brings about new knowledge and a change to grow"; and "By reviewing the evidence and developing our concept map, we integrated research to promote evidence-based practice for our patients."

THE PROCESS OF USING CONCEPT MAPPING AND SIMULATION IN UNDERGRADUATE EDUCATION

A similar process for undergraduate education can be implemented to include faculty-led didactic information, development of a student group concept map, simulation activity, debriefing, and on-line or face-to-face examinations. The level of intensity for undergraduate education can be initiated early in the program to include vital signs and physical appraisal and progress to simulators with complex, multisystem organ failure. In this university setting, one of the simulation rooms is designed as an individual's home. Students in their community health rotation can be exposed to a home assessment before engaging in a live home clinical visit. For all scenarios, the students would be expected to follow the clinical practice guidelines with the level of evidence provided. The differences for undergraduate education are related to student roles, such that there would be 2 professional nurses, one unlicensed personnel, and a family member. Using these roles allows for interprofessional collaboration and nurse/patient/caregiver communication.

THE PROCESS OF USING CONCEPT MAPPING AND SIMULATION FOR HOSPITAL STAFF DEVELOPMENT/ANNUAL COMPETENCY-BASED EDUCATION

Staff development and annual competency-based education would benefit from the aforementioned model so as to provide the participants with an immersive experiential format for learning. Staff nurses would be exposed to clinical competencies via a Web-based course, assigned to groups to develop a concept map, and to prepare for the simulation experience. Hospital educators would be trained to facilitate the learning experience as previously discussed. Competency-based education using concept mapping and simulation would enhance nurses' skill set, assessment, and intervention strategies, with resultant improvement in patient outcomes.

SUMMARY

Concept mapping and simulation provide professional nurses in the academic and practice environment with an opportunity for experiential learning. This integral combination allows for learning to be congruent with the national clinical practice guidelines that support and promote nurse-sensitive indicators. Implications for practice are forthcoming as data are collected on the impact on health outcomes when using concept mapping and simulation.

REFERENCES

1. American Nurses Association. Nursing: scope and standards of practice. Silver Spring (MD): Nursesbooks.org; 2010.
2. Institute of Medicine. The future of nursing: leading change, advancing health. Washington, DC: The National Academies Press; 2011.
3. Institute of Medicine. Crossing the quality chasm: a new health system for the 21st century. Washington, DC: National Academics Press; 2001.
4. Albanese M, Evans D, Schantz C. Engaging clinical nurses in quality and performance improvement activities. Nurs Adm Q 2010;34(3):226–45.
5. Doran D. Preface. In: Doran D, editor. Nursing sensitive outcomes: state of the science. Sudbury (MA): Jones and Bartlett; 2003. p. viii.
6. National Quality Forum. National Voluntary Consensus Standards for Nursing Sensitive care Performance Measure Set Maintenance. Available at: http://www.qualityforum.org/Projects/n-r/Nursing-Sensitive-CareMaintenance.aspx. Accessed July 22, 2013.
7. Spross J, Lawson M. Conceptualization of advanced practice nursing. In: Hamric A, Spross JA, Hanson CM, editors. Advanced practice nursing an integrative approach. 4th edition. St Louis (MO): WB Saunders; 2009. p. 33–74.
8. Lasater K. Clinical judgment development. Using simulation to create an assessment rubric. J Nurs Educ 2007;46(11):496–503.
9. Finkelman A, Kenner C. Provide patient-centered care. In: Professional nursing concepts competencies for quality leadership. 2nd edition. Burlington (MA): Jones and Bartlett; 2013. p. 265–99.
10. Rowles CJ, Russo BL. Strategies to promote critical thinking active learning. In: Billings D, Halstead J, editors. Teaching in nursing a guid for faculty. 3rd edition. St Louis (MO): Saunders; 2009. p. 238–61.
11. Novak J. Meaningful learning for empowerment. In: Novak J, editor. Learning, creating and using knowledge. New York: Erlbaum; 1998. p. 19–34.
12. Braungart M, Braungart R, Gramet P. Applying learning theories to healthcare practice. In: Bastable S, editor. Nurse as educator principles of teaching and learning for nursing practice. 4th edition. Burlington (MA): Jones and Bartlett; 2014. p. 63–110.
13. Muirhead B. Creating concept maps: integrating constructivism principles into online classes. In: International Journal of Instructional Technology Distance Learning. 2006. Available at: http://itdl.org/journal/jan_06/article02.htm. Accessed January 10, 2010.
14. Gul R, Boman J. Concept mapping: a strategy for teaching and evaluation in nursing education. Nurse Educ Pract 2006;6:199–206.
15. Distler JW. Critical thinking and clinical competence: results of the implementation of student-centered teaching strategies in an advanced practice nurse curriculum. Nurse Educ Pract 2006;7:53–9.
16. Wells H, Kinchin I. Quantitative and qualitative measures of student learning at the university level. Stud High Educ 2008;56:221–39.
17. Novak J, Gowin D. Concept mapping for meaningful learning. In: Learning how to learn. New York: Cambridge University Press; 1984. p. 15–54.
18. Duffy J. Nosocomial infections: important acute care nursing-sensitive outcome indicators. AACN Clin Issues 2002;13(3):358–66.
19. Del Bueno D. A crisis in critical thinking. Nurs Educ Perspect 2005;26:278–82.
20. Jeffries P. A framework for designing, implementing, and evaluating simulations used as teaching strategies in nursing. Nurs Educ Perspect 2008;26(2):96–103.

21. Decker S, Sportsman S, Puetz L, et al. The evolution of simulation and its contribution to competency. J Contin Educ Nurs 2008;39(2):74–80.
22. Kolb D. The process of experiential learning. In: Kolb D, editor. Experiential learning: experience as the source of learning and development. New Jersey: Prentice-Hall; 1984. p. 38.
23. American Association of Colleges of Nursing/John A. Hartford Foundation. Adult-gerontology acute care nurse practitioner cocmpetencies. Washington D.C. 2012.

A Nursing Focus on EMR Usability Enhancing Documentation of Patient Outcomes

Cecilia Anne Kennedy Page, DNP, RN-BC, CPHIMS, PMP[a],*,
Aric Schadler, PhD(ABD)[b]

KEYWORDS

- Usability • Usability checklist • User interface design • Efficiency • Effectiveness
- Satisfaction

KEY POINTS

- Nursing practice requires a focus on the usability of technology, such as the electronic medical record, to enhance patient outcomes.
- Usability is a critical dimension of health information technology design to support human responses in the use of information in clinical decision making.
- Integration of the usability checklist as a standard tool in the software design process and user acceptance testing is a method to strive for safe technology in health care.

INTRODUCTION

Health Information Technology (Health IT) makes it possible for health care professionals to more effectively manage patient care through secure use and sharing of health information. The Health Information Technology for Economic and Clinical Health Act passed in 2009, a part of the American Recovery and Reinvestment Act, is an incentive program designed to expedite the adoption of an electronic medical record (EMR) by 2014.[1] The provisions of the Health Information Technology for Economic and Clinical Health legislation focus on utilizing this infrastructure with the underlying aim of promoting population health through meaningful use of EMRs as opposed to a focus on technology alone.[2] Over the next 2 to 3 years, adoption of EMRs into clinical practice settings will be rapid as reimbursement becomes linked to meaningful use of these systems and the ultimate tracking of clinical conditions or outcomes to promote health.

Implementing electronic health records without a focus on usability is the largest barrier to widespread adoption of EHRs.[3] Broadly defined, usability is viewed as the

[a] Information Technology Services, University of Kentucky HealthCare, 900 South Limestone Street, Charles T. Wethington Building, Suite 317, Lexington, KY 40536-0200, USA;
[b] Information Technology Services, 2333 Alumni Plaza, Suite 110, Lexington, KY 40517, USA
* Corresponding author.
E-mail address: cecilia.page@uky.edu

Nurs Clin N Am 49 (2014) 81–90
http://dx.doi.org/10.1016/j.cnur.2013.11.010
0029-6465/14/$ – see front matter © 2014 Elsevier Inc. All rights reserved.

capacity of a system to allow users to carry out their tasks safely, effectively, efficiently, and enjoyably.[4] The International Standards Organization defines usability as "the effectiveness, efficiency, and satisfaction with which the intended users can achieve their tasks in the intended context of product use."[5] In essence, a system with good usability is easy to use, effective, intuitive, forgiving of mistakes, and allows the user to perform necessary tasks quickly.[6] In the context of nursing health care IT or the adoption of the electronic health record, usability addresses the capability of a nurse to perform tasks associated with care delivery.

Achieving the health care reform goals of broad EMR adoption and meaningful use will require that the usability of these systems in nursing practice be addressed. There is a direct relationship between usability and clinical productivity, error rates, user fatigue, and user satisfaction. All of these are critical indicators of poor usability.[6] With the rapid deployment of EMRs, usability evaluations can identify design features of health information technology that pose a risk for influencing patient safety.[7] However, these evaluations are not commonly performed and early adopters did not integrate usability evaluations as a part of standard design and implementation. This integration was not considered because early adopters focused on adoption rather than on usability. Nursing practice requires a focus on the usability of technology, such as the EMR, to embed features of usability within the tool to enhance patient outcomes and optimal utilization by the end-user.

BACKGROUND

The goal of health care technology utilization is to promote a safer and more efficient system of care. In a recent publication by the Committee on Patient Safety and Health Information Technology of the Institute of Medicine (IOM),[8] health IT is presented as a positive enabler to transform the way health care is delivered. The inherent risk is that health IT adds complexity to an already complex health care system. Inappropriately designed and applied health IT may lead to unintended adverse consequences and errors.[8] From a sociotechnical model view, technology is approached as interactive with the people, processes or workflow, organization, and environment as key factors that influence the success of health IT outside of the technology itself[9] and this becomes the foundation for understanding the user-technology interaction. This relationship must be considered in a usability evaluation and approach for understanding how the user integrates technology into their daily practice in the provision of safe care.

The user-centered design principle is considered a "bedrock principle" for creating usable systems and devices.[5] In the current information age, health care providers are challenged with managing an increasing amount of information now presented in an electronic modality.[10] To assimilate the vast influx of information, user-centered design methods must be taken into consideration to design and create systems. These methods result in systems that are easy to learn, increase user productivity and satisfaction, increase user acceptance, decrease user errors, and decrease user training time.[10] User-centered design methods include tasks and goals of the users, functional analysis of cognitive activities of the users, user analysis of the characteristics of the users, environmental analysis of the environments in which the users work, and the representational analysis of the manner in which information displays to the users.[10] It is the workflow and cognitive processing for the users that warrants consideration in the system design. This focus embraces the users and shifts the cognitive work to the patient processes and away from just the mechanics of the EMR system. Software design and its effect on workflow, as well as an effective user interface, are key determinants of usability.[8]

Integration of user-centered design strategies is a fundamental requirement of health IT development and effective integration into complex work systems. The conceptual model of usability is depicted in **Fig. 1**. Usability principles designed into the user interface should simplify work processes, resulting in improved efficiency, effectiveness, and satisfaction. Effectiveness in usability is viewed as the degree to which an interface facilitates users accomplishing their tasks or goals.[5] Effectiveness is measured by the quality of the documentation, error rates, or outcome data.[5] Efficiency is measured by the length of time required to complete a task and how easy the system is to use. Efficiency is measured by time performing particular tasks, the number of clicks, screen movement, or process measurement.[5] For the end-user, usability is a determinant of performance. Good usability will allow the user to perform the expected task faster and more efficiently.[11]

Satisfaction is a person's subjective response to his/her interaction with a system.[5] Satisfaction is measured through survey results, subjective comments, or feedback on system use. Enhanced usability demonstrated through efficiency, effectiveness, and satisfaction metrics will enhance the adoption of the technology, meaningful use of the system, and enhanced patient outcomes.

The Institute of Medicine (IOM) report contended that poor usability is one of the single greatest threats to patient safety but, once improved, usability can be an effective promoter of patient safety.[8] The IOM report also endorsed usability guidelines by stating that health IT should make it easy to do the right thing by the providers in care delivery processes. Usability focuses on the aim of right information in the right place for the right clinician at the right time. It is critical for usability principles to be integrated into the EMR to promote adoption and, more importantly, meaningful use of this technology. The ever-increasing usability of health IT systems will be a key enabler to achieving population health.

In 2011, the Agency for Healthcare Research and Quality released a publication promoting an EHR tool kit aimed at addressing the lack of understanding of the cognitive needs of clinicians that result from common problems in human-computer interactions.[12] Health IT applications must be designed, developed, and evaluated with serious considerations of the characteristics of the users, their tasks, and their environments.[12] Clinicians continually process complex data, information, and knowledge to support a range of activities from diagnosis, care planning, treatment, and health management. Usability issues impacting the clinician cognitive ability include, but

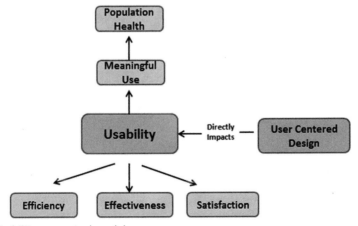

Fig. 1. Usability conceptual model.

are not limited to, (1) poor organization and display of information from limited screen space and poor interface design; (2) interference with practice workflow from a lack of alignment with workflow patterns of clinicians; (3) increases in cognitive burden from massive amounts of information demands while remaining accurate and efficient in a time constrained work day; and (4) poor design of system functions at the point of care from excessive use of defaults, alerts, copying forward, and other system configurations.[12] Each of these designs effect usability of the EMR and do not adequately support the mental models of the clinicians, resulting in the increased opportunity for errors and resistance to EMR adoptions.

User testing provides feedback as to what extent people can actually perform the intended functions of a system design. When this step is omitted, the users complain that the software does not support their basic requirements and this initiates a cycle of dissatisfaction and error-prone designs.[13] Consequences may include frustrated users, decreased efficiency coupled with increased cost, disruptions in workflow, and increases in health care errors.[14] When an organization deploys EMRs or new functionality required in process improvements in health care settings, usability testing must be a component part of the deployment for adoption and success.

At the University of Kentucky Healthcare, the journey to roll-out of the EMR began with the deployment of computerized physician/provider order entry in 2004 and clinical documentation in the patient care settings in 2008. Both of these functionalities were implemented in an instant changeover approach across the enterprise. In 2012 the organization found the system was wrought with opportunities for improvement. The end-user satisfaction was poor as demonstrated through staff surveys and verbal complaints in staff forums held with senior management. Monitoring of the nurse-sensitive outcome indicators demonstrated a below benchmark performance in quality metrics. Adoption of the EMR was required through an organizational mandate but poor design had resulted in poor utilization and ineffective use of the EMR. In 2012, the division of nursing championed an initiative focused on the usability of the EMR as a strategic priority.

METHODOLOGY/STUDY DESIGN

The aim of this initiative was to increase the efficiency, effectiveness, and satisfaction of the nursing interface with the IT system to enhance the nursing influence in optimizing patient outcomes. This work spanned 2 years and required a full redesign of the clinical documentation to ensure the system met the nursing requirements for a usable system. The approach was divided into 4 phases in order to focus on the various patient populations and nursing care delivery models in these clinical areas. Phase 1 included the medical-surgical and critical care adult populations; phase 2 focused on the obstetric and neonatal populations. Phase 3 included the pediatric population, and the final phase was centered on behavioral health patient populations. The Emergency Department was initially designed with the usability principles and did not require the full redesign focus. The ultimate requirement in each patient population was a system that made it easy to tell the patient story and reflect evidence-based nursing practice.

Integral to the design was the engagement and input from the nurses. One of the most common reasons systems are poorly designed is that the users are not engaged in the design and testing of the systems. Users must be engaged early and throughout the design phase of development to complete incremental design-test cycles until an accepted prototype is established.[5] This approach guided the development of this project and front-line nurses were engaged through every phase of this project. The project lifecycle used as the framework for project management is depicted in **Fig. 2**. The phases of plan, design, build, test, activate, and outcomes were replicated for each phase of the project. During this design process, formative usability activities were carried out in support of defining the software capability, understanding the user and user workflow, and making iterative improvements to the product.[6] Iterative design sessions followed the cognitive flow of the nurse in the clinical settings and guided the development of the documentation according to usability attributes.

The design phase of this project included coordinating these iterative design sessions to obtain requirements from the nursing work teams. These teams were responsible for gathering the requirements for clinical documentation in support of evidence-based practice for these patient populations. As the clinical experts, the leadership relied on these individuals to provide a critical analysis of best practices. An assessment of current state workflow was completed before the initiation of design sessions. Design sessions were conducted with each design group to include the development of the future state workflow for nursing process documentation in each of these patient populations and the system design characteristics. A prototype was developed as a part of the formative review process for future state work and design sign-off. On completion of the prototype, user acceptance testing occurred integrating the usability checklist into the review process. Each task in the future state workflow was evaluated according to the identified attributes of usability.

Fundamental to the project approach was the development of a usability checklist to guide the system designs. During the design process, formative usability activities were carried out in support of defining the software capability, understanding the user and user workflow, and making iterative improvements to the product.[6] Iterative design sessions followed the cognitive flow of the nurse in the clinical settings and guided the development of the documentation according to usability attributes. The checklist developed by the Health Information Management Systems Society Usability Task Force[6] was adopted and modified adding error monitoring for the identification of safety parameters in particular.[15] The usability checklist depicted in **Fig. 3** was used in the design phase to guide decisions ensuring the system configuration reflected the nursing cognitive thought processes and workflow. During the testing phase, the usability checklist followed the workflow and tasks of the end-users as patient care scenarios to evaluate screen design and data flow. Defects were identified with a usability focus and any elements that scored a 3 or 4 were considered serious usability errors and required resolution before moving forward. This checklist provided an alternative view in the configuration of data to ensure information was intuitive to facilitate critical thinking, not hinder.

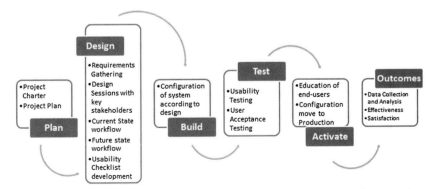

Fig. 2. System development life cycle utilized as the project management framework.

Usability Checklist

Please rate your experience with the software design by completing the following checklist when you have finished entering the patient scenarios.
Please rate the attribute in the box to the right according to how you feel the task met that principle design. Place a check if it meets the criteria, otherwise, rate 1-4 as defined below.

	Process / Workflow	Task to be Completed	Simplicity	Visibility	Minimalist	Naturalness	Consistency	Memory	Cognition	Feedback	Flexibility	Language	R gentation	Error Free	Comments
1	Based on the phase of care such as admission, shift assessment, procedure, education, plan of care, discharge, transfer, or other workflow by the nurse.	Evaluation is based on the task to be completed by the clinician in this scenario													
2															
3															
4															
5															
6															
7															
8															
9															
10															

Usability Attributes

Simplicity	Lack of visual clutter; Concise information display
Visibility	Appropriate feedback and display of information
Minimalist	Less is more. Contains only pertinent information and avoids
Naturalness	Familiarity and ease of use;Common terminology; Flows with user
Consistency	Learnability – matches experience with other systems; internal
Memory	Minimize requirement for user to memorize a lot of information to
Cognition	Presents the information needed for the task at hand; do not need to
Feedback	Informative feedback. Prompts and informative feedback given for
Flexibility	Allows users to customize and utilize shortcuts in order to accelerate
Effective use of language	Concise, unambiguous, standard, approved terminology (no use of unapproved abbreviations)
Effective presentation	Density – 80% of screen is meaningful / Color – meaningful to user (red, yellow, green) / Readability –scan quickly with high comprehension
Error Free	Completion of tasks without errors

Score	Rating	Description
0	No problem	Not a usability problem
1	Cosmetic	Does not need fixing unless extra time is available
2	Minor usability	Fixing-low priority. No impact on patient safety -
3	Major usability	Fixing-High priority. Patient safety impact & nurse
4	Usability	Imperative to fix. Severe patient safety and nurse

Date: _____   Printed Name: _____

Signature: _____

Fig. 3. Modified usability checklist adopted from the Health Information Management Systems Society Usability Task Force.

The project phase 1, adult medical surgical and critical care, and phase 2, obstetrics and neonatal intensive care, are completed at the time of this publication. Phase 3, pediatrics, was implemented and in the final stage of data collection, while phase 4, behavioral health, was under design. The documentation is pertinent specifically to the patient population served.

RESULTS

Table 1 reflects a summary of the outcome statement reflecting the attributes of satisfaction, effectiveness, and efficiency. Phase 1, medical-surgical and critical care populations, successfully tracked effectiveness measurement through nurse-sensitive indicator metrics. Phase 2, obstetrics and neonatal intensive care populations, successfully tracked efficiency measurement through time study analysis. Both phases 1 and 2 tracked satisfaction measurement through a survey methodology.

Documentation of patient outcomes is reflected in the nursing assessment within the patient medical record. Nursing-sensitive indicators reflect the structure, process, and outcomes of nursing care.[16] Patient outcomes that are determined to be nursing sensitive are those that improve if there is a greater quantity or quality of nursing care. Effectiveness metrics were measured through the aggregate patient outcomes for 3 key nursing-sensitive indicators: catheter-associated urinary tract infections (CAUTI), pressure ulcer presence, and restraint utilization. These metrics are most heavily influenced by nursing documentation for compliance to nursing protocols, integration of evidence into practice, and alternative nursing measures to reduce incidence. The pre- and postmetrics (6 months pre- and post-) for CAUTI rate decreased 30%, whereas the indwelling catheter days in these units only altered 1.6%. Documentation of the presence of pressure ulcers, stages I to IV, demonstrated a significant decline of 43.8%. Finally, restraint utilization demonstrated a 14.3% decrease. Standardization and simplicity of the documentation fields in the record enabled more accurate documentation of patient condition and care delivered.

In the efficiency metrics, the keystroke level analysis measured human performance and interaction with the system. A matched-pairs design was used, matching the pre- and postmeasures on the case scenarios, the nurse, the documents entered, and the environment (same room, computers, and time of day). The analysis of this information was computed into a paired t-test using SPSS® v21.[17] Most significant was the time to complete a process or segment identified in the workflow. The results showed an average time of 12 minutes 48 seconds (0:12:48.10) to complete a document in the preusability environment, compared with only 7 minutes 1 second (0:07:01.26) in the postusability environment, a 45.2% decrease in documentation time. This time was a highly significant decrease with a p value of .00005. This value was directly attributed to the elimination of major free text fields and open-ended documentation areas as well as a decrease in redundant documentation requirements.

Satisfaction was measured using the computer system usability questionnaire (CSUQ),[18] a nonproprietary computer-based interface measurement tool. This tool measures the system usefulness, informational quality, and interface quality. The overall CSUQ's coefficient α is 0.95. The tool is a 12-question, 7-point Likert scale format ranging from strongly disagree to strongly agree. This test was administered in a pre- and post- format to compare the baseline satisfaction with the current system design with the satisfaction levels of the system postusability. The postsurvey was circulated 30 to 60 days after the usability changes using an electronic push to the end-user nursing community. The design for the presurvey administration was at the start of the education session before any changes were described to the staff

Table 1
Outcome analysis demonstrating satisfaction, effectiveness, and efficiency benefits

| Outcome | Attribute | Evaluation Tool | Metric | Measurement | | Results—% |
				Pre	Post	Change
Increase staff satisfaction with use of the redesigned EMR	Satisfaction	CSUQ	Adult Med Surg/Critical Care	50.6	55.5	9.8%
			OB/NICU	48.0	58.9	22.6%
Improve quality measure outcomes for Nurse Sensitive Indicators	Effectiveness	Nursing Analytics report for 3 nurse-sensitive indicators: CAUTI, Pressure Ulcers, and Restraints (6 mo pre/post)	CAUTI (no. reported)	127	88	30.70%
			CAUTI (rate)	4.532	3.191	29.60%
			Foley days	28,019	27,570	1.60%
			Pressure ulcers	617	347	43.80%
			Restraint days	6001	5241	12.70%
			Restraint %	5.89%	5.05%	14.30%
Decrease time and redundancy in documentation tasks	Efficiency	Keystroke-level model; program = AutoIt Mouse Recorder (recorder utility)	Time study by document/process (OB/Peds)	12.48	7.01	45.20%

nurse. To summarize the entire survey, each survey was given a total score comprising the sum of the Likert Scale question responses. Thus, if someone marked "Strongly Agree" for all 12 questions, that survey would have scored an 84, or if they had marked "Strongly Disagree" for each question, the survey would have scored a 12. For phase 1, there were 1525 respondents (n = 1014 pre; n = 511 post) with a preusability survey total score average of 50.6, compared with a postusability score of 55.5, an overall positive reflection of satisfaction increasing 9.8% (P- value <.0001). Phase 2 reflected 267 respondents (n = 188 pre; n = 79 post) with a preusability survey total score average of 48.0, compared with a postusability score of 58.9, an overall positive reflection of satisfaction increasing 22.6% (P- value <.0001). These results reflect an increase in end-user satisfaction postusability redesign.

DISCUSSION AND IMPLICATIONS

The outcomes of this project were statistically significant. The outcomes of efficiency, effectiveness, and satisfaction were all improved with the redesign of the EMR focusing on usability principles. Several strengths of this study included the engagement of the staff nurses in each phase of the project from planning and design through testing and activation. The staff believed they owned the design because it was the analysis of their workflow and integration of evidence into practice that drove the configuration and challenged the status quo. The cognitive flow was simplified to follow the thought processes of the nurse in the assessment and implementation of care at the bedside. Fundamentally, this project focused on the impact of technology on the workflow and cognition of the end-users, the nurses.

The adoption of technology will continue to be the cornerstone in the transformation of health care in the twenty-first century. The rapid deployment of the EMR speaks to the need for a focus on usability to ensure the infrastructure supports an environment that is safe, timely, equitable, efficient, and patient-centered.[15] This study demonstrated the tremendous influence usability of an electronic system has on the clinicians using the technology. Designing systems with an inherent focus on workflow, simplicity, cognition, visibility, feedback of information, presentation of data, and other principles of usability is critical to driving enhanced patient outcomes. The use of a usability checklist to ensure design and testing according to these attributes should become standard in the system development lifecycle. These results demonstrate to a high degree of sensitivity the linkage between usability principles and efficiency, effectiveness, and satisfaction of an EMR. The users of the system are more satisfied, demonstrate better patient outcomes, and have time back as providers of patient care.

SUMMARY

Usability is a critical dimension of a health IT system. Implementing a focus on usability provides the interaction for human responses to interpret and ultimately use information in clinical decision-making. To improve care and outcomes, information systems must work well for the people who use them. Overall, the goal in the EMR is to use the technology in a way that can be executed effectively, efficiently, safely, and with optimal user satisfaction while capturing the needed clinical documentation.

Integration of the usability checklist as a standard tool in the software design process and user acceptance testing is a method to strive for safe technology in health care. Designing usable technology for complex domains is difficult work but yet there is a call to action to ensure the systems being installed today are providing a safe platform for care tomorrow.

REFERENCES

1. American Recovery and Reinvestment Act, H.R. Res., 111th Cong., TITLE XIII (2009) (enacted).
2. Bluementhal D, Tavenner M. The "meaningful use" regulation for electronic health records. N Engl J Med 2010;363(6):501–4.
3. HIMSS Usability Task Force. Promoting usability in Health Organizations: Initial steps and progress toward a healthcare usability maturity model [White paper]. 2011. Available at: www.HIMSS.org. Accessed February 23, 2013.
4. Kushniruk AW, Patel VL. Cognitive and usability engineering methods for the evaluation of clinical information systems. J Biomed Inform 2004;37:56–76. Available at: http://dx.doi.org/10.1016/j.jbi.2004.01.003.
5. Schumacher RM, Lowry SZ. NIST Guide to the processes approach for improving the usability of electronic health records. National Institute of Standards and Technology; 2010. NISTIR 7741.
6. HIMSS EHR Usability Task Force. Defining and testing EMR usability: principles and proposed methods of EMR usability evaluation and rating [White paper]. 2009. Available at: www.HIMSS.org. Accessed February 23, 2013.
7. Russ AL, Weiner M, Russell AA, et al. Design and implementation of a hospital-based usability laboratory: insights from a Department of Veterans Affairs laboratory for health information technology. Jt Comm J Qual Patient Saf 2012;38(12):531–9.
8. Committee on Patient Safety and Health Information Technology, Institute of Medicine. Health IT and patient safety. Washington, DC: The National Academies Press; 2012.
9. Sittig DF, Singh H. A new sociotechnical model for studying health information technology in complex adaptive healthcare systems. Qual Saf Health Care 2010; 19(Suppl 3):i68–74. Available at: http://dx.doi.org/10.1136/qshc.2010.042085.
10. Johnson CM, Johnson TR, Zhang J. A user-centered framework for redesigning health care interfaces. J Biomed Inform 2005;38:75–87. Available at: http://dx.doi.org/10.1016/j.jbi.2004.11.005.
11. Abran A, Khelifi A, Suryn W. Usability meanings and interpretations in ISO standards. Software Qual J 2003;11:325–38.
12. Agency for Healthcare Research and Quality. EHR usability toolkit: a background report on usability and electronic health records [Web-based toolkit]. 2011. Available at: www.AHRQ.gov. Accessed March 16, 2013.
13. Johnson CW. Why did that happen? Exploring the proliferation of barely usable software in healthcare systems. Qual Saf Health Care 2006;15:i76–81. Available at: http://dx.doi.org/10.1136/qshc.2005.016105.
14. Yen P, Bakken S. Review of health information technology usability study methodologies. J Am Med Inform Assoc 2012;19(413422). Available at: http://dx.doi.org/10.1136/amiajnl-210-000020.
15. Office of the National Coordinator for Health information Technology. Health information technology patient safety action and surveillance plan. 2013. Available at: www.healthit.gov. Accessed March 16, 2013.
16. American Nurses Association: NursingWorld (2013), Nursing-Sensitive Indicators. Available at: www.nursingworld.org. Accessed March 23, 2013.
17. IBM Corp. Released 2012. IBM SPSS Statistics for Windows, Version 21.0. Armonk, NY: IBM Corp.
18. Lewis R. IBM computer usability satisfaction questionnaires: psychometric evaluation and instructions for use. Int J Hum Comput Interact 1995;7(1):57–78.

Using a Web-based Patient-Provider Messaging System to Enhance Patient Satisfaction Among Active Duty Sailors and Marines Seen in the Psychiatric Outpatient Clinic: A Pilot Study

Jane J. Abanes, DNP, RN, PMHCNS, PMHNP[a],*,
Susie Adams, PhD, RN, PMHNP[b]

KEYWORDS

- Web-based messaging • On-line communication • Patient satisfaction • Psychiatry
- Military

KEY POINTS

- In recent years, mental disorders among service members resulted in significant health care and occupational burden.
- Change is needed in successfully implementing patient improvement initiatives; however, change can only be achieved by engaging the participation of patients, clinicians, governing bodies, policymakers, researchers, and others.
- Patient satisfaction is vital to the practice of psychiatry and remains one of the key indicators of whether the delivery of mental health care is adequate.
- Implementing a secure communication system, in addition to face-to-face engagement, has a potential to improve the 21st century health care system and help promote safe, effective, patient-centered, timely, efficient, and equitable mental health care.
- The impact of stressors experienced in the military has led to a surge of active duty service members seeking help through mental health services.

INTRODUCTION

In recent years, mental disorders among service members resulted in significant health care and occupational burden.[1] From the years 2000 to 2011, there were

The authors have nothing to disclose.
[a] Department of Mental Health, Naval Health Clinic Hawaii, 480 Central Avenue, JBPHH, HI 96860, USA; [b] Psychiatric Mental Health Nurse Practitioner Program, Vanderbilt University School of Nursing, 384 Frist Hall, 461 21st Avenue South, Nashville, TN 37240, USA
* Corresponding author.
E-mail address: Jane.abanes@med.navy.mil

936,283 active duty military members who were diagnosed with at least one mental health disorder. In 2011, mental disorders were the leading cause of hospital admissions of service members in the United States.[2] Nevertheless, clinical actions have been progressively slow in integrating ways to increase patient satisfaction in mental health care. As the demands for mental health services increase, patients, providers, and researchers are calling for more ways to increase patient satisfaction, enhance patient communication, and improve mental health outcomes. Change is needed in successfully implementing patient improvement initiatives; however, change can only be achieved by engaging the participation of patients, clinicians, governing bodies, policymakers, researchers, and others.

As the 21st century health care continues to evolve, patients and providers are becoming more computer-savvy in accessing and providing care. This pilot study investigates the use of a Web-based messaging asynchronous system to increase patient satisfaction in a psychiatric outpatient setting. The availability of a secure communication medium will be available in addition to 15-minute medication management or brief supportive psychotherapy appointments. Albeit brief follow-up appointments are short and concise, they often require members to be away from their work spaces for longer periods of time. Although face-to-face appointments are still recommended at least monthly, psychiatric patients may ask questions, request to schedule appointments, or request medication refills in between face-to-face interactions. Patient satisfaction is vital to the practice of psychiatry and remains one of the key indicators of whether the delivery of mental health care is adequate. The patient's involvement in decision-making could lead to improved treatment outcomes.[3] Patient satisfaction may have direct influence on patient adherence to treatments.[4] Successfully addressing the patient's concerns, fears, and threats creates a sense of fulfillment not only to the patient but also to the clinicians as well. When patients are satisfied with the care they receive, clinicians are generally happier and more fulfilled. Consequently, a cascade of positive events transpires wherein clinicians become better caregivers for their patient, which then fosters more patient satisfaction. Enhancing the use of technology in health care could help reduce patient harm, decrease health care cost, and maximize scarce resources.[5] Implementing a secure communication system, in addition to face-to-face engagement, has a potential to improve the 21st century health care system and help promote safe, effective, patient-centered, timely, efficient, and equitable mental health care.[6]

The impact of stressors experienced in the military has led to a surge of active duty service members seeking help through mental health services. However, the demands for increased services can exacerbate an already overwhelmed system. Because of the shortage of well-trained providers and the increased administrative workload, the mental health outpatient clinic is unable to meet the demands for more appointments. Wait times to receive initial appointments and the average gap between follow-up visits is about 3 to 4 weeks. As a result, many patients have become dissatisfied with their care. Patients complain that their providers are not able to effectively meet their needs through traditional modes of interaction such as face-to-face or via a telephone call because of the limited availability of appointments. Telephone consults about medication inquiries have increased to an average of 4 per day per provider. Navigating through the system to schedule appointments, request for medication refills, or simply ask a question has become burdensome because the service member plays "phone tag," competes for parking, and takes time away from work to visit the clinic. Such logistical inconveniences, to spend an average of 15 minutes to see a provider for medication management, could result in patient dissatisfaction among those who are already suffering from mental illness. In response to the increasing needs of mental health services, in the outpatient psychiatric setting, one additional psychiatric provider and then a third provider was added within the past year. As an additional resource, this article investigates the use of a Web-based patient-provider messaging system to increase patient satisfaction in the psychiatric outpatient clinic.

BACKGROUND

Barriers to providing effective mental health interventions to Sailors and Marines include shortage of well-trained mental health providers, provider burnout, and stigma of receiving mental health care in the military. Throughout the Department of Defense (DoD), shortages of mental health providers is a relevant concern.[7] In light of the increased burden of mental health problems as a result of the Overseas Contingency Operations (OCO), the Department of the Navy's goal is to conduct 100% predeployment and postdeployment health screenings of personnel-assessing for medical, mental health, and psychosocial issues. Postdeployment screenings are conducted every 3 months, 6 months, 12 months, and then 18 months consecutively by a Licensed Independent Practitioner. The goals of deployment screenings are to detect psychological ailments and to refer service members who may need further medical or mental health consultation.[8] Required screenings could result in increased referrals to outpatient mental health and could potentially overwhelm available resources. In addition, rapid turnovers among military personnel are common. Military providers could be deployed and may be temporarily assigned to another location for months at a time. Because of the increased prevalence of traumatic stress disorders that exist among their patient population, mental health providers who treat military personnel are more prone to burnout.[9] Military providers may have been exposed to traumatic experiences themselves or suffer from surmounting occupational stressors as they fulfill the demands of being providers as well as officers. Provider burnout can lead to ambivalence, reduced job performance, attrition, poor self-care, and suicide.[9]

To tackle the burden of mental disorders, the Pentagon allocates approximately 2 billion dollars to the DoD's mental health[10] and 2.9 billion dollars to the Veteran's Health Administration (VHA) annually for mental health and substance abuse services.[11] Services were rendered to approximately 1 million veterans from years 2005 to 2007.[11] The financial burden of mental health problems does not address the human cost. Since 2001, 2676 American troops have died by suicide.[10] The suicide rate soared to 18% in 2012—averaging one active duty U.S. soldier committing suicide each day.[10] Over the last 12 years, diagnosis of mental health disorders in the military has increased to 65% in which common diagnoses consist of adjustment disorders, depressive and anxiety disorders, and posttraumatic stress disorders.[2] Particularly, military behavioral health clinics commonly diagnose and provide interventions to service members with adjustment disorders.[1] After 6 months of receiving a mental health disorder diagnosis, the attrition rate from military service is 27% of the 1.5 million of all active duty service personnel including Army, Air Force, Navy, and Marines who received mental health care in 2000.[1] Veterans seen in 16 VHA facilities increased from 5.02 million in 2005 to 5.20 million in 2008. Among those veterans, those who were diagnosed with mental health disorders increased from 1.45 million to 1.69 million. Among the veterans who received care from 2005 to 2008, suicide rates differed by age. The higher suicide rate was associated with VHA users older than 30 years compared with those younger than 30 years who received VHA services and with those who did not seek care at the VHA.[12]

The problem of homelessness among veterans has been widely delineated through various investigations. Seventeen percent of the nation's homeless adults surveyed from 47 communities are reported as veterans.[13] Individuals 30 to 40 years old who were discharged from military service with psychiatric difficulties and substance abuse problems are found to be at higher risk for homelessness or exacerbation of mental illness.[14] The extent of mental health problems experienced by military service members significantly affects their caregivers as well. Military caregivers are the spouses, parents, children, colleagues, and friends or anyone who provides care for a person with physical or mental illnesses.[15] Military caregivers perform a myriad of roles to support their loved ones including health assistance, case management, mental and emotional support, and legal, financial, and advocacy roles. The complexity of these roles may lead to the caregiver's health deterioration, mental and emotional distress, isolation, and loss of income. Nevertheless, despite the burdensome effects of caregiving, a limited amount of resources is available or services remain uncoordinated for military caregivers.[15]

The burden of mental health problems and consequences of Operation Enduring Freedom and Operation Iraqi Freedom have sparked national interest, particularly the alarming increase in suicide rates among active duty servicemen and newly discharged veterans. The media's attention and government's push to increase availability of behavioral services to military personnel has significant implications because the military is the second largest employer in the United States. In 2011, there were over 2 million active duty, Reservists, and National Guard servicemen in the United States.[16] To continue to support and defend the United States, the military organization is essential to the nation's security: "As the Navy look to the future, the morale and welfare of the nation's Sailors, their families, and the service's civilian work force, will continue to be a central concern".[17]

Literature Review of the Concept of Patient Satisfaction

The pursuit of quality health care began when the Institute of Medicine's (IOM's) Council issued a white paper, "America's Health in Transition: Protecting and Improving Quality," in 1994. The white paper highlighted the conclusion that "quality can and must be measured, monitored, and improved."[18] IOM posits that one of the ways to measure the outcome of health care services is by determining the patient's satisfaction with the care received. In the last decade, there has been an abundance of interest in implementing a patient-centered approach to health care and empowering patients to take charge of their own health. A paradigm shift in health care has emerged wherein practitioners are no longer the authorities in determining the treatment plan; instead, patients become the experts and main collaborators in the decision-making process. Consequently, a question was raised of whether the quality chasm approach may be applied to mental health care, an infrastructure with unique characteristics and volatile dynamics. The experts concluded that the quality framework could indeed be effectively applied to mental health and substance abuse problems. Most importantly, the experts highlighted that patient preference prevails in the treatment of mental health conditions.[19] The IOM's first recommendation for organizations to improve the 21st Century Health Care System is to continually reduce the burden of illness and to improve the health and functioning of health care consumers. As a way to translate this general statement into more specific, manageable health care objectives, the IOM has developed 6 aims: safe, effective, patient-centered, timely, efficient, and equitable.[6] This paper integrates these 6 essential aims in the definition of patient satisfaction. Patient satisfaction happens when patients receive safe and effective care, timely and efficient service, patient-centered treatment approach, and respectful and confidential patient interactions (**Fig. 1**).

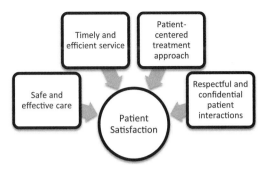

Fig. 1. Patient satisfaction concept. (*Data from* the Institute of Medicine's (IOM). Crossing the quality chasm: a new health system for the 21st century. Washington, DC: National Academy Press; © 2001.)

Appraisal of Literature Regarding Web-Messaging Between Patient-Provider

According to a survey, a total of 69% of 2000 adults use a computer at work, home, or other location, and 81% of computer users go on-line.[20] Another survey data indicate that 40% of the 1000 respondents expressed frustration that they have to physically visit the office to ask their physicians simple questions. Most importantly, 57% of respondents expect that the Internet will likely reduce or eliminate their frustrations regarding health care.[21] The Office of the National Coordinator for Health Information Technology created under the Bush administration has set the goal of nationwide adaptation and use of Electronic Health Records by 2014. Shortly after his first inauguration, President Barack Obama signed into law the American Recovery and Reinvestment Act of 2009, providing $19.2 billion for health information technology.[22] An increasing body of evidence indicates that patients and providers are embracing the use of on-line communication as a way to communicate about their health status and treatment strategies.[23] The advancement of technology has sparked considerable interest in the adaptation of Electronic Health Records to improve health outcomes. However, the explosion of on-line communication has mostly spread across the primary care arena. Secure Web-messaging in the primary care has been associated with positive patient response,[24–26] decreased office visits, improved measurable outcomes, and exceptional patient satisfaction.[27] Physician attitudes in the use of a secure Web-based portal remain positive.[28] Currently, there are no reported studies that describe or investigate the effectiveness of a Web-based messaging system within a psychiatric outpatient setting. The mere possibility that confidentiality and privacy may be breached when unintended users accidentally access patient records significantly contributes to an agency's reluctance to adopt a computerized patient portal in psychiatry.[29] However, "the best window on the safety and quality of care is through the eyes of the patient."[6] Health care organizations should continuously develop ways of responding to the patient's needs thoroughly and timely, and beyond face-to-face visits, such as the use of Internet.[6]

METHODS

The purpose of this pilot study was to determine the effectiveness of a Web-based patient-provider messaging system in enhancing patient satisfaction among active duty Sailors and Marines with services received in a psychiatric outpatient clinic. Naval Health Clinic Hawaii (NHCH) uses *RelayHealth* by RelayHealth Corporation of Emeryville, California as its computerized patient portal within the primary care clinics.

RelayHealth is designed to improve the coordination of care between clinic providers and hospitals.[30] *RelayHealth* is an electronic communication system that allows users, including patients, providers, and ancillary staff, to experience asynchronous messaging as well as obtain educational resources. Patients are able to obtain various nonurgent services on-line, such as request to schedule or cancel an appointment, request for laboratory tests or results, request renewal of prescriptions, request referrals, or simply ask the provider or office staff a variety of nonurgent questions. The site requires patients to register and log-in with a password. Messages are only accessed by the registered provider and authorized front office staff. Web-site security is achieved with 128-bit Secure-Socket-Layer and a secure server.[30]

Study Design

The pilot study was a part of a process improvement initiative that was ongoing in the psychiatric outpatient clinic. Patients were asked to complete pre- and postsurveys using the DoD's on-line Internet-based and Health Insurance Portability and Accountability Act compliant Interactive Customer Evaluation Survey.[31] Data were collected retrospectively on satisfaction scores from the surveys before implementation of the Web-based messaging system and then compared them with the same satisfaction scores after implementation. A request for an Institutional Review Board (IRB) waiver of consent as well as an exemption to IRB protocol to access the survey data was submitted to Vanderbilt University and Navy Medicine West for Human Subject Protection. On approval of IRB, 53 subjects were recruited during the preimplementation phase. A nonrandomized presurvey and postsurvey were used for the pilot study. Baseline surveys were completed on March 1, 2013 until June 19, 2013. The initial stages of presurveys were conducted as part of an ongoing quality improvement project. The Web-based patient-to-provider system was piloted within a 12-week period from June 19, 2013 to September 11, 2013. Reminders for patient satisfaction repeat surveys were sent via *RelayHealth* at least monthly after initiation.

Setting and Subjects

All subjects were active duty service members seen by the Psychiatric Mental Health Nurse Practitioner (PMHNP) in Naval Health Clinic, Hawaii. The first 50 patients seen by the PMHNP, except those who have severe psychosis or complex personality disorder, were invited to participate in the study. On approval by the PMHNP, those who registered via *RelayHealth* received e-mail notification of their participation in the system. In this pilot study, the PMHNP was the only psychiatric provider registered to have access to *RelayHealth* along with 6 psychiatric technicians who were trained to use the Web-messaging system for a minimum of 1 hour. A *RelayHealth* NHCH Champion consistently monitored activities to facilitate services for providers, staff, and patients. Patients were treated for a variety of psychiatric disorders including mood, anxiety, and personality disorders. Some patients had comorbid alcohol use-related diagnoses. Treatments were mainly medication management, supportive psychotherapy, and acupuncture. Other than the implementation of the computerized portal, there were no other changes to the clinic routine. Most patients were stable on medication and continued to work as active duty service members. Patients who had a history of psychotic disorder or had active psychosis and those who have complex personality disorders were excluded from the sample population.

Data Collection Tools

Patient satisfaction surveys were available electronically via the Interactive Customer Evaluation Survey on-line. Hand-out instructions were provided to patients on how to fill out the on-line survey. Most items on the survey questions consisted of a 5-point Likert scale response set. At the end of the survey, participants were asked to provide additional feedback. Open-ended questions were included such as "Comments and Recommendations for Improvement." The surveys did not include any Personally Identifiable Information or Personal Health Information. The results of the presurveys were used as baseline information on patient satisfaction and were reviewed retrospectively. After 1 month of the initial implementation of the study, and at least monthly thereafter, patients were reminded via *RelayHealth* to complete repeat survey questionnaires on-line. On completion of the study, a retrospective review and collection of satisfaction scores were conducted.

Data Analysis

Descriptive statistics were used to interpret data obtained from satisfaction scores.

RESULTS

Among the 53 patients who were invited to register within the 12-week pilot study, the total number of patients who enrolled in the Relay Health Communication System (RHCS) was 33. Seventeen of the 33 enrolled patients initiated messages yielding a 52% utilization rate. Twenty of the 33 enrolled patients completed the on-line postsurvey, yielding a response rate of 60%. A total of 340 messages were collated among the front office staff, provider, and patients; of these, 81 were initiated by patients. One hundred percent of patients' inquiries were responded by the provider or front office staff within 48 hours. **Table 1** shows preintervention and postintervention average ratings of use of phone system and patients' overall satisfaction. **Figs. 2–4** show the number of initiated messages by patients per day of the week. **Fig. 2** depicts Wednesdays as having the highest messaging activity during the initial implementation of the system; subsequently, messages peaked on Thursdays throughout implementation as shown in **Figs. 3** and **4**. **Table 2** shows a summary of the total number of messages per day of the week and the associated percentages for each day over 81 total messages initiated by patients.

Preintervention Results

Presurvey showed an 85% average satisfaction rate of the ease of appointment by phone system, 81% satisfaction rate with the time it took the clinic to return the phone calls, and 98% satisfaction rate that NHCH met the needs and expectations of safe, quality patient care and service. The baseline study showed a 92% approval rate with patient overall satisfaction level with NHCH.

Table 1
Patient perception of services. Pre- and postimplementation of RHCS

Standard Scale Questions	Preintervention Average Rating	Postintervention Average Rating	Change in Mean Score
Ease of appointment by phone system	4.3 (n = 14)	4.1 (n = 21)	(0.2)
Time clinic return phone call	4.1 (n = 14)	4.2 (n = 19)	0.1
NHCH met patient expectations	4.9 (n = 14)	5.0 (n = 14)	0.1
Patient overall patient satisfaction	4.6 (n = 15)	4.8 (n = 15)	0.2

( ) Indicates decrease in mean score.

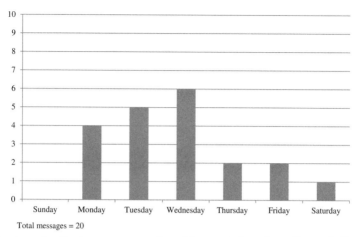

Total messages = 20

Fig. 2. Number of patient messages per day of the week from June 19 to July 23.

Postintervention Results

Postsurvey showed 82% average satisfaction rate of the ease of appointment by phone system, 84% satisfaction rate with the time it took the clinic to return the phone call, and 100% satisfaction rate that NHCH met the needs and expectation of safe, quality patient care and service. The postsurvey study showed a 96% overall satisfaction rate with NHCH. **Table 1** illustrates a decline in the average rating of the ease of phone system, whereas the average rating for overall patient satisfaction slightly increased with the use of the Web-messaging system. As **Table 3** portrays, 21% (4/19) of responders used the RHCS "more than 3 times," 5% (1) "3 times," 26% (5) "twice," 32% (6) once, and 16% (3) never. Fifty-six percent (10/18) were overall "very satisfied" with RHCS; 33% (6) were "satisfied," and 11% (2) were "neutral." Of patients, 78% (14/18) reported that the provider responded "within 24 hours" using RHCS, 17% (3) "within 48 hours," 6% (1) "no response." The "no response" likely indicates the patient who did not use RHCS as the *RelayHealth* system report indicated

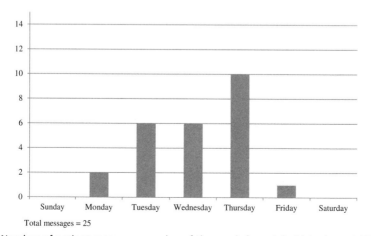

Total messages = 25

Fig. 3. Number of patient messages per day of the week from July 24 to August 23.

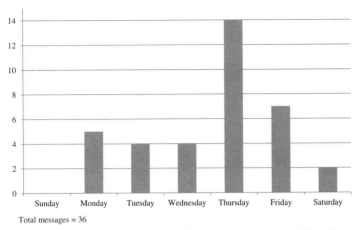

Total messages = 36

Fig. 4. Number of patient messages per day of the week from August 24 to September 11.

that 100% of messages were responded by the provider within 72 hours. Sixty-five percent (13/20) were overall "very satisfied" with Web-messaging compared with the phone system, 25% (5) were "satisfied," and 10% (2) were neutral. Seventy-four percent (14/19) of patients rated the respectfulness and confidentiality of interactions with provider and staff as "very satisfied," 21% (4) as "satisfied," and 5% (1) as "neutral." Sixty-one percent (11/18) rated the ease of use and navigation of RHCS as "very satisfied" and 39% (7) rated the ease of use and navigation of RHCS as "satisfied." **Box 1** highlights positive experiences of patients regarding RHCS.

DISCUSSION

In this pilot study, patients reported overall satisfaction using a secure on-line system when communicating with their provider in the psychiatric outpatient clinic. Many responders rated the Web-based messaging system more satisfactory than the phone system. Services that patients mostly used on-line were requesting medication refills, requesting appointment cancellation, or rescheduling and asking nonurgent questions about their medications or other concerns. Patients found the system easy to use and were satisfied with their provider's response time. Most users communicated with their provider on Thursdays. Anecdotal reports from provider and front office staff implied convenient use of the system. In addition, they reported that on-line

Table 2		
Patients' pattern of use of RHCS		
Day of the Week	**Number of Messages**	**% (n = 81)**
Sunday	0	0
Monday	11	14
Tuesday	15	18
Wednesday	15	18
Thursday	27	33
Friday	10	12
Saturday	3	4

Table 3
Patient perceptions of RHCS

Standard Scale Questions	Multiple Choice Questions	% of Responses
Patient utilization of RHCS (n = 19)	Four or more times—4	21
	Three times—1	5
	Two times—5	26
	Once—6	32
	Never—3	16
Overall satisfaction with RHCS (n = 18)	Very satisfied—10	56
	Satisfied—6	33
	Neutral—2	11
	Dissatisfied—0	0
	Very dissatisfied—0	0
Time until provider response using RHCS (n = 18)	Within 24 h—14	78
	Within 48 h—3	17
	Within 72 h—0	0
	Within 1 wk—0	0
	No response—1	6
Patient rating of RHCS compared with previous phone system (n = 20)	Very satisfied—13	65
	Satisfied—5	25
	Neutral—2	10
	Dissatisfied—0	0
	Very satisfied—0	0
Patient rating of RHCS of respectfulness and confidentiality (n = 19)	Very satisfied—14	74
	Satisfied—4	21
	Neutral—1	5
	Dissatisfied—0	0
	Very satisfied—0	0
Ease of use for RHCS (n = 18)	Very satisfied—11	61
	Satisfied—7	39
	Neutral—0	0
	Dissatisfied—0	0
	Very satisfied—0	0

messaging between provider and patient as well as between provider and front office staff decreased "phone tag" and reduced time and effort filling out telephone request forms or typing telephone consults to provider. Most of these results were consistent with the report of Liederman and colleagues[25] on their primary care study that the use of Web-based messaging system improved patient satisfaction, increased staff

Box 1
Patient comments regarding RHCS

- This is an easy way to communicate and check in with my doctor. We both have very busy schedules and if I have a question or I need more refills on my prescription, it is perfect to just send a message. I don't know why this hasn't been done before.

- I have not used *RelayHealth* with my current provider, but I have used it in the past. I like it better than the traditional method of playing phone tag with the provider.

- The *RelayHealth* system is amazing. The interaction and availability of interaction with the provider are beyond words. This system needs to be brought fully on-line for all providers and nurses. This system has the potential to cut man hours drastically on answers that can be provided to patients at home.

efficiency, and reduced clerical work.[32] Front office staff that experienced some difficulty logging-in during the initial stages of the system's implementation was less active in using the system. Meanwhile, staff members who were proficient right at the beginning of the project remained proactive throughout system implementation. The provider's as well as the staff's active engagement in responding to patients on-line may have had a positive influence on the patients overall experience. Psychiatrists were previously reluctant to communicate with patients on-line for fear of possible breach of security and confidentiality but with adequate education and training of providers, staff, and patients, such barriers could be averted. Providers were also concerned that workload will increase as patient messages surge the system's in box. On the contrary, patient messages averaged about 7 per week per provider.

LIMITATIONS

Because this was a pilot study, the sample size of the provider, staff, and patients was considerably small; therefore, it is difficult to say that this is a representative sample of the demographics studied. Some patients stationed on ships were prone to deploy several times per year or month, which may have contributed to a low survey response rate. Surveying the participants on-line had some advantages and disadvantages. Having an on-line survey ensured anonymity of patients; however, patients were less inclined to fill out surveys using their home computers because of other responsibilities or distractions and were reluctant to use their work computers for patient privacy reasons. The study did not quantitatively measure provider and staff perception regarding the system or obtain telephone volume. The patient satisfaction survey had some limitations. Multiple choice answers such as "no response" should be replaced by "not applicable" for the question on provider's response time. The question about "respect and confidentiality" should not be limited to one question to accurately rate patient's perception on these areas.

SUMMARY

The availability of a secure on-line communication system in the psychiatry clinic offered patients a convenient way of interacting with their provider. Having this accessibility contributed to patient satisfaction. Increased accessibility and satisfaction may alleviate the patient's stress level while waiting to see the provider in the office. Patient's timely communication with the provider may also facilitate treatment interventions. Provider and front office staff's regular use of the system is essential in ensuring success of the Web-messaging. Further research should explore effects of the secure on-line communication system to patient satisfaction, patient stress level, clinic no-show rates, provider and staff satisfaction and productivity, access to care, and the number and time staff and providers spend on patients calls.

ACKNOWLEDGMENTS

LCDR Jane J. Abanes would like to acknowledge the following individuals who assisted in conducting the study: CAPT Connie Stamateris; Kimberly Dubois, RN; LCDR Megan Rieman; Ms. Susan Fukuda; Ms. Nemy Membrere; CDR Traci Brooks; CDR Ruchira Densert; and CDR Dennis Spence. The views expressed in this article are those of the authors and do not necessarily reflect the official policy or position of the Department of the Navy, Department of Defense, nor the U.S. Government.

REFERENCES

1. Garvey Wilson AL, Messer SC, Hoge CW. U.S. military mental health care utilization and attrition prior to the wars in Iraq and Afghanistan. Soc Psychiatry Psychiatr Epidemiol 2009;44:473–81.
2. Armed Forces Health Surveillance Center. Mental disorders and mental health problems, active component, U.S. armed forces, 2000–2011. MSMR 2012; 19(6):11–7.
3. Clever SL, Ford DE, Rubenstein LV, et al. Primary care patients' involvement in decision-making is associated with improvement in depression. Med Care 2006;44(5):398–405.
4. Dang BN, Westbrook RA, Black WC, et al. Examining the link between patient satisfaction and adherence to HIV care: a structural equation model. PLoS One 2013;8(1):1310–71.
5. Weingart SN, Simchowitz B, Padolsky H, et al. An empirical model to estimate the potential impact of medication safety alerts on patient safety, health care utilization, and cost in ambulatory care. Arch Intern Med 2009;169(16):1465–73.
6. Institute of Medicine. Crossing the quality chasm: a new health system for the 21st century. Washington, DC: National Academy Press; 2001.
7. Jones MD, Etherage JR, Harmon S, et al. Acceptability and cost-effectiveness of military telehealth mental health screening. Psychol Serv 2012;9(2):132–43.
8. Deployment Health Clinical Center. Enhanced post-deployment health assessment (PDHA) process (DD Form 2796). Available at: http://www.pdhealth.mil/dcs/dd_form_2796.asp. Accessed July 14, 2012.
9. Ballenger-Browning KK, Schmitz KJ, Rothacker JA, et al. Predictors of burnout among military mental health providers. Mil Med 2012;176(3):253–60.
10. Thompson M, Gibbs N. The insidious enemy: why the pentagon is losing the war against military suicide. Time 2012;180(4):22–31.
11. Greenberg GA, Rosenheck RA. An evaluation of an initiative to improve Veterans Health Administration mental health services: broad impacts of the VHA's mental health strategic plan. Mil Med 2009;174(12):1263–9.
12. Katz IR, McCarthy JF, Ignacio RV, et al. Suicide among veterans in 16 states, 2005 to 2008: comparisons between utilizers and nonutilizers of Veterans Health Administration (VHA) services based on data from the National Death Index, the National Violent Death Reporting System, and VHA administrative records. Am J Public Health 2012;102(1):105–10.
13. National survey of homeless veterans in 100,000 homes campaign communities. Available at: http://www.va.gov/HOMELESS/docs/NationalSurveyofHomelessVeterans_FINAL.pdf. Accessed March 6, 2013.
14. Goldstein G, Luther JF, Jacob AM, et al. A preliminary classification system for homeless veterans with mental illness. Psychol Serv 2008;5(1):36–48.
15. Tanielian T, Ramchand R, Fisher MP, et al. Military caregivers: cornerstones of support for our nation's wounded, ill, and injured veterans. Available at: www.rand.org. Accessed March 12, 2013.
16. Kelley ML, Jouriles EN. An introduction to the special section on U.S. military operations: effects on military members' partners and children. J Fam Psychol 2011; 25(4):459–60.
17. Navy program assessment. Available at: http://www.navy.mil/navydata/policy/vision/vis98/vis-p05.html. Accessed July 19, 2012.
18. Institute of Medicine. America's health in transition: protecting and improving quality. A statement of the council of Institute of Medicine. Available

at: http://www.nap.edu/openbook.php?record_id=9147&page=1. Accessed September 22, 2013.

19. Institute of Medicine. The national roundtable on health care quality: measuring the quality of health care. Available at: http://www.nap.edu/catalog/11470.html. Accessed November 20, 2012.

20. Harris Interactive. P.C. and internet use continue to grow at record pace, according to Harris interactive survey. Available at: http://harrisinteractive.com/news/allnewsbydate.asp?NewsID=55. Accessed February 2, 2013.

21. Taylor H, Leitman R. Study reveals big potential for the internet to improve doctor-patient relations. Available at: http://harrisinteractive.com/news/newsletters/healthnews/HI_healthcarenews-v1-issue1.pdf. Accessed February 2, 2013.

22. Steinbrook R. Health care and the American recovery and reinvestment act. Available at: http://www.nejm.org/doi/full/10.1056/NEJMp0900665. Accessibility verified February 2, 2013.

23. Katz SJ, Moyer CA. The emerging role of online communication between patients and their providers. J Gen Intern Med 2004;19(9):978–83.

24. Hassol A, Walker JM, Kidder D, et al. Patient experiences and attitudes about access to a patient electronic health care record and linked web messaging. J Am Med Inform Assoc 2004;11(6):505–13.

25. Liederman E, Morefield C. Web messaging: a new tool for patient-physician communication: original investigation. J Am Med Inform Assoc 2003;10(3): 260–70.

26. Volk LA, Pizziferri L, Wald J, et al. Patients' perceptions of a Web portal offering clinic messaging and personal health information. AMIA Annu Symp Proc 2005;1147.

27. Baer D. Patient-physician e-mail communication: the Kaiser permanente experience. J Oncol Pract 2011;7(4):230–3.

28. Kittler AF, Carlson GL, Harris C, et al. Primary care physician attitudes towards using a secure web-based portal designed to facilitate electronic communication with patients. Inform Prim Care 2004;12(3):129–38.

29. Lamberg L. Confidentiality and privacy of electronic medical records: psychiatrists explore risks of the "information age". JAMA 2001;285(24):3075–6.

30. RelayHealth. Available at: http://www.relayhealth.com/about-us/corporate-overview. Accessed February 2, 2013.

31. ICE (Interactive Customer Evaluation) survey. Available at: http://ice.disa.mil/. Accessed May 14, 2013.

32. Liederman EM, Lee JC, Baquero VH, et al. Patient-physician web messaging. The impact on message volume and satisfaction. J Gen Intern Med 2005;20(1): 52–7.

A Critical Analysis and Adaptation of a Clinical Practice Guideline for the Management of Behavioral Problems in Residents with Dementia in Long-Term Care

Nanette Lavoie-Vaughan, MSN, ANP-C, DNP*

KEYWORDS

- Clinical practice guideline • Dementia • Behavioral problems • Long-term care

KEY POINTS

- Studies show that up to 75% of patients with dementia have behavioral problems.
- Because of the current public concern about the use of antipsychotics for patients with dementia, treatment must be based on evidence-based data.
- As the number of persons with dementia continues to grow and the burden on long-term care staff to provide safe and quality care increases, evidence-based data must be used to develop individualized plans of care.

INTRODUCTION

According to experts, all persons with dementia will develop a behavior problem or a personality change as the disease progresses.[1,2] Studies show that up to 75% of patients with dementia have behavioral problems.[3,4] Clinical practice guidelines to assist health care providers in managing difficult behaviors have been developed by the American Psychiatric Association,[5] American Geriatrics Society (2012),[6] Group Health Cooperative,[7] University of Iowa Gerontological Nursing Interventions Research Center,[8] and American Medical Directors Association.[9]

STATEMENT OF THE PROBLEM

Clinical practice guidelines exist for the management of long-term care (LTC) residents' behavioral problems. However, the most commonly referenced guidelines

College of Nursing- Graduate Program, East Carolina University, Health Sciences Building Greenville, NC 27858, USA
* 3819 Donna Road, Raleigh, NC 27604.
E-mail address: nursenan1@earthlink.net

Nurs Clin N Am 49 (2014) 105–113
http://dx.doi.org/10.1016/j.cnur.2013.11.006
0029-6465/14/$ – see front matter © 2014 Elsevier Inc. All rights reserved.

detail protocols for psychotropic medication, but lack behavioral interventions other than 2 main categories: redirection and distraction.[10,11] These categories do not take into consideration the residents' individual needs and the applicability to the environment. Seldom, if ever, are implementation issues such as staff education and buy-in mentioned in the guidelines. Without staff that is trained to perform behavioral interventions, the plan will not succeed.[12] This scholarly project focused on these deficits.

PURPOSE

The purpose of this scholarly project was to critically analyze and adapt guidelines for managing behavioral problems of residents in LTC facilities and to draft an adaptation for implementation in the author's practice. The adaptation focused on individualizing interventions derived from evidence-based research and included strategies for maximize staff buy-in and implementation. The overall goal was to decrease the use of psychotropic medications, particularly antipsychotics, and develop an evidence-based clinical practice guideline to assist providers in meeting that goal.

BACKGROUND AND SIGNIFICANCE

The incidence of dementia is increasing in the United States. This project focused on the nurse practitioner practice in 2 states: North Carolina and Tennessee. The behavioral problems associated with dementia often prompt psychiatric consultations, which result in residents being prescribed psychotropic medications (**Table 1**).[13]

Nurse practitioners providing psychiatric consultation face many challenges. First, the administration of psychotropic medications in LTC facilities has the potential to result in deficiencies in federal regulation F222, which addressed chemical restraints, and F329, concerning unnecessary medications.[14] The U.S. Food and Drug Administration[15] has extended black box warnings to all classes of antipsychotic medications that were found to cause increased risk of death in elderly patients with dementia. Because of the current public concern about the use of antipsychotics for patients with dementia, evidence-based data must be used to determine treatment.[16]

Secondly, behavioral problems are a complex issue that is influenced by the biology of the disease, the environment in which the resident resides, psychosocial factors, and the staff's knowledge and expertise in managing the behavior. Lovheim and colleagues[17] identified that men more often exhibited aggressive and regressive behavior, wherein women more often exhibited depressive behavior. No differences between the sexes were noted for passiveness and hallucinations. Researchers have suggested the importance of assessing medical conditions, environment, medications, and other causes as a source of behavioral problems, and implementing an individualized plan of care incorporating behavioral interventions.[3,4,13,18–23] Pain,

Table 1 Statistics related to targeted population of study		
Demographic	With Alzheimer Disease in Long-Term Care	With Behavior Problems
United States	43% older than age 85 y	—
North Carolina	89,223	80%–90%
Tennessee	70,494	80%–90%
Total	159,737	127,769+

Data from Alzheimer's Association Report. Alzheimer's disease facts and figures. Alzheimers Dement 2012;8:131–68. Available at: http://www.alz.org/downloads/facts_figures_2013.pdf.

infection, fear, loneliness, medication side effects, or anxiety may cause behavioral issues.[24] Cohen-Mansfield[25] suggests that behavior in patients with dementia is often an attempt to signal that a need is not being met, an effort to get needs met directly, or a sign of frustration. She identifies 4 types of behavior:

1. Reaction to stressful situations
2. Wandering and interfering with normal activities
3. Failure to inhibit actions, thoughts, and emotions
4. Mismatch between the person and the environment

Lastly, aggressive behavior continues to challenge and burden the staff of LTC facilities. Working in an LTC facility is associated with a higher risk of physical or verbal assault.[26] Staff require education and support to deal with these behaviors safely and efficiently. As many LTC facilities institute person-centered care and an ability-focused approach to care planning, the nurse practitioner must refer to an evidence-based clinical practice guideline to treat behavioral problems.[27]

SYNTHESIS OF EVIDENCE

An online search of professional organizations and guideline collection Web sites was conducted to locate pertinent clinical practice guidelines. Only those applicable to patients with dementia were selected (those from the American Psychiatric Association,[5] American Geriatrics Society (2011),[6] Group Health Cooperative,[7] University of Iowa Gerontological Nursing Interventions Research Center,[8] and American Medical Directors Association[9]). The selected guidelines were analyzed using the Appraisal of Guidelines for Research and Evaluation (AGREE) checklist (AGREE Trust, 2012),[28] and the American Medical Directors Association guideline was chosen.

A comprehensive literature review of evidence-based literature and research was conducted on CINAHL, PubMed, and Evidence-Based Medicine Reviews using the key words "dementia," "behavior," and "interventions." A total of 200 articles were obtained and sorted by level of evidence. Emphasis was placed on articles from the past 5 years. A further search was performed to narrow the focus to specific interventions using the key words "bright light therapy," "Montessori," "aromatherapy," "massage," "therapeutic touch," "pet therapy," "music therapy," and "activities." This search yielded 159 articles.

Data collected included those on assessment and treatment of behavioral problems and specific interventions for behavior modification, environmental interventions, alternative therapies, and distraction techniques. Meta-analyses and systematic reviews were evaluated using Preferred Reporting Items for Systematic Reviews and Meta-Analyses (PRISMA),[29] and randomized-control studies were evaluated with Consolidated Standards of Reporting Trials (CONSORT).[30] The author selected 82 articles for the development of the guideline after approval from the clinical team, which was composed of a psychiatrist, 2 nurse practitioners in psychiatric practice in LTC, and the author. The articles deleted included studies with low scores on the PRISMA and CONSORT, those with predominantly anecdotal or case studies, and those with strictly opinions. The goal was to use studies with levels of evidence of 1 through 4 on the hierarchy of evidence scale, and an A or B rating on the Strength of Recommendation Taxonomy (SORT) evidence rating system. Close to 50% of the studies were on alternative therapies, and a quarter of those were conducted outside the United States. Most of the studies were on music therapy and aromatherapy, and most had small sample sizes, with a need for replication. Other interventions included games, pet therapy, swing glider use, Snoezelen multisensory rooms, massage, and light.

The remaining studies highlighted staff approach and education, distraction and redirection, and environmental changes. All of these studies were limited by small sample size, and some were limited by minimal effect.

In consultation with the clinical team, the interventions were chosen based on the strongest supporting data. This practice supports the future plans to have the guideline adopted for use and replicate the studies for those interventions used most by staff. These plans are outside the scope of this project.

CONCEPTUAL AND THEORETICAL FRAMEWORK

This project is serving as a springboard for behavior management for a significant portion of the LTC population. The project incorporated concepts related to behaviors, nursing practice, and adaptation. A framework to include these concepts had to be multilayered and address each of the concepts individually and as a whole. Furthermore, the framework considered the complexity of the project population: patients with dementia who had behavioral problems. The theory/framework addresses the antecedents of challenging behavior and how it relates to the planned interventions. The 2 theories/frameworks used were Wiedenbach's[31] *The Helping Art of Nursing* and the Progressively Lowered Stress Threshold (PLST) model.[32]

Wiedenbach's Helping Art of Clinical Nursing

The 2 tenets of Wiedenbach's[31] theory are

1. Nursing skills are performed to achieve a specific patient-centered purpose rather than just for the sake of performing the skill itself
2. Whatever an individual does at any given moment represents the best available judgment for that person

Wiedenbach defines an individual as anyone who is receiving help, instruction, or advice from a member of the health care profession. She further defines the need for help as "any measure desired by the patient or his/her caregiver that has the potential to restore or to extend the ability to cope with various life situations that affect health and wellness."[31(p54)]

Wiedenbach's theory is supported by components of a nursing philosophy, a prescriptive theory, and a practice model. The underlying nursing philosophy speaks to

- A reverence for life,
- Respect for dignity,
- Autonomy,
- The individuality of each human being, and
- A resolution to act personally and professionally on held beliefs.

The prescriptive theory focuses on a central purpose for meeting the needs of patients, which the practitioner uses in clinical practice; a prescription or guideline for the fulfillment of the central purpose; and the realities of the immediate situation that influence the central purpose. The practice model begins with observation of the presenting behavior, followed by exploration of the meaning and cause of the behavior, and determining the patient's ability to resolve the behavior with help from the health care professional.[31(p54-57)]

This theory mirrors the purpose for clinical practice guidelines for behavior management. The practice model is similar to the methods recommended for determining the cause of the behavior and being able to intervene properly.[33] It incorporates all

3 concepts of this scholarly project and is based on the science of nursing. The framework focuses on the underlying reason for behavior and how it can be managed.

Progressively Lowered Stress Threshold Model

The PLST model proposes that, "with disease progression, individuals experience increasing vulnerability and a lower threshold to stress and external stimuli."[32(p399)] PLST suggests that minimizing environmental demands that exceed functional capacity and regulating activity and stimulation levels throughout the day can reduce agitation. Specific factors include the physical environment (auditory and visual stimulation), the social environment (communication style of caregivers, influence of other residents), or factors that are modifiable but are internal to the individual (pain, fatigue, medical conditions).

Boltz and colleagues[34] identified the essentials of care for behavioral problems related to the PLST model:

1. Maximize safe function: use familiar routines, limit choices, provide rest periods, reduce stimuli when stress occurs, and routinely identify and anticipate physical stressors (eg, pain, urinary symptoms, hunger, thirst).
2. Provide unconditional positive regard: use respectful conversation, simple and understandable language, and nonverbal expressions of touch.
3. Use behaviors to gauge activities and stimulation: monitor for early signs of anxiety (pacing, facial grimacing) and intervene before behavior escalates.
4. Teach caregivers to listen to behaviors: monitor language pattern (repetition, jargon) and behaviors (rummaging) that might show how the person reduces stress when needs are not being met.
5. Modify the environment: assess the environment to assure safe mobility, and promote way finding and orientation through cues.
6. Provide ongoing assistance to the caregiver: assess the need for education and support.

These essentials were used as a template for selecting behavioral interventions for the adapted guideline.

APPLICATION OF THEORY AND FRAMEWORK

The theory and framework define the purpose of clinical practice guidelines for behavior management. They also acknowledge the role of nursing art and science in helping patients with behavioral problems, and support the underlying causes of behavior that need to be addressed. In understanding the relationship among stress, environment, and behavior and staying true to nursing's roots of caring, a clinical practice guideline was drafted to provide individualized and appropriate behavioral interventions.

Wiedenbach's nursing theory meshes with the complex issues of behavioral problems and the underlying tenets of this guideline. The theory speaks to the residents whose actions at any given moment are a response to their environment and their interactions with others. This response is especially evident in persons with behavioral problems. One of the purposes of this guideline is to provide interventions that are specific to the individual and have the potential to restore or extend the individual's ability to cope. Wiedenbach's practice model is the basis for assessment and treatment of behavioral problems, because it outlines the need to find the trigger or antecedent, explore the possible causes, and individualize the treatment.

The PLST model speaks to the potential causes of behavior: physical environment, social environment, and modifiable conditions. Assessment of each of these areas is needed to develop and implement appropriate interventions. Bolt's (2012) essentials of care related to the PLST model can be applied to the types of interventions that were selected for use in the guideline. The first essential, to maximize safe function, is addressed in the interventions that reduce stimuli, anticipate needs, and establish consistent routines. Specific interventions include

- Sensory enhancement,
- Relaxation,
- Music,
- Aromatherapy,
- Structured activity, and
- Pet therapy.

The second essential, to provide unconditional positive regard, is addressed in the interventions related to staff education and training on proper approaches to residents and communication skills. The third essential, to use behavior to gauge activity and stimulation, is addressed in the assessment phase of treatment and reflected in all of the behavioral interventions.

The fourth essential, to teach caregivers to listen to behaviors, is addressed in the staff educations interventions of communication training, approach to residents, and techniques for working with residents with dementia. The fifth essential, to modify the environment, is addressed in the environmental interventions:

- Light therapy
- Monitoring systems
- The creation of a home-like environment

The sixth essential, to provide ongoing assistance to the caregiver, is the process of evaluation to determine which interventions are working, which are not, and where further training and education is needed.

The theory and framework were the initial starting points for the development of this guideline. A review for consistency was performed when the interventions were selected, revised, and accepted. A final analysis was performed at the completion of the guideline.

METHODOLOGY
Needs Assessment

The need for a clinical practice guideline for behavior management was identified by the author at the time of employment with a national psychiatric practice in January 2012. This concern was validated by other nurse practitioner staff in North Carolina and Tennessee during a monthly staff meeting. It was proposed that this author, with the assistance of the clinical team, draft a clinical practice guideline.

Project Design

The methodology for this scholarly project followed the steps of the adaptation process for clinical improvement.[35] These steps are

- To search existing guidelines,
- Assess the guidelines for quality,
- Assess the applicability of the recommendations to the target setting,
- Perform a literature review,
- Adapt the guideline, and
- Implement the adapted guideline.

The first step was to find guidelines that were applicable to residents with dementia in LTC. The AGREE checklist was completed on the selected guidelines, and consensus was reached on which guideline to adapt. The articles gathered were critically analyzed using the PRISMA, CONSORT, and evidence-rating scales. Once again, consensus was reached on which interventions to include in the guideline. The guideline was drafted and reviewed for final acceptance.

Resources

The primary resources were library databases, secondary forms of evidence, and the knowledge and expertise of the clinical team. The project took 6 months to complete, with a total cost of $800 for travel and copying fees. The use of Internet search engines and Skype facilitated the gathering of data and discussions with colleagues.

PROJECT RESULTS

The completion of this scholarly project resulted in an evidence-based guideline for behavior management of LTC residents with dementia. This guideline is applicable for any provider in LTC, but especially for those providing psychiatric consultation. It contains

- Assumptions,
- Definitions,
- Levels of evidence,
- Recognition of behavioral problems,
- Sample documentation,
- Assessment of problems,
- Treatment,
- Specific interventions (eg, sensory enhancement and relaxation, structured activity, social contact, environmental changes, therapies),
- Staff education, and
- Monitoring.

APPLICABILITY TO ADVANCED PRACTICE

Nurse practitioners are playing a pivotal role in the care of LTC residents. The doctor of nursing practice has the additional education and expertise to develop and implement evidence-based clinical practice guidelines for critical issues in this vulnerable population. The number of residents with dementia will increase as the population ages, and the need for best practices for care will increase with that need.

Evidence-based interventions are available for the nonpharmacologic management of dementia-related behavioral problems. However, replication of these studies is needed to continue to support this clinical practice guideline. Dissemination of the guideline and education of providers and staff can be accomplished through the publication of the guideline and presentation at professional conferences. All of these tasks are easily in the purview of advanced practice nursing.

SUMMARY

As the number of persons with dementia continues to grow and the burden on LTC staff to provide safe and quality care increases, evidence-based data must be used to develop individualized plans of care. The nurse practitioner plays a pivotal role in this process through disseminating information, doing research, and assisting staff in formulating care plans. Although individualizing every plan may be difficult, an evidence-based guideline may make the process easier for the practitioner.

REFERENCES

1. Ballard CG, Gauthier S, Cummings JL, et al. Management of agitation and aggression associated with Alzheimer disease. Nat Rev Neurol 2009;5(5): 245–66.
2. Koppel J, Goldberg TE, Gordon ML, et al. Relationships between behavioral syndromes and cognitive domains in Alzheimer disease: the impact of mood and psychosis. Am J Geriatr Psychiatry 2012;20:994–1000.
3. Desai AK, Grossberg GT. Recognition and management of behavioral disturbances in dementia. Prim Care Companion J Clin Psychiatry 2001;3(3): 93–109.
4. Gauthier S, Cummings J, Ballard C, et al. Management of behavioral problems in Alzheimer's disease. Int Psychogeriatr 2010;22(3):346–72.
5. American Psychiatric Association. Treatment of patients with Alzheimer's disease and other dementias, second edition. Available at: http://psychiatryonline.org/content.aspx?bookid=28&sectionid=1679489. Accessed March 1, 2012.
6. AGS viewpoint: use of pain control decreased agitation by 17%. Ann Longterm Care 2012. Available at: http://americangeriatrics.org. Accessed March 1, 2012.
7. Group Health. Dementia and cognitive impairment: diagnosis and treatment guideline. Available at: www.ghc.org/all-sites/guidelines/dementia.pdf. Accessed November 8, 2013.
8. McGonigal-Kenny ML, Schutte DL. Nonpharmacologic management of agitated behaviors in persons with Alzheimer disease and other chronic dementing conditions. J Gerontol Nurs 2006;32(2):9–14.
9. American Medical Directors Association. Clinical practice guidelines in the long term care setting. Available at: http://www.amda.com/tools/guidelines.cfm. Accessed November 8, 2013.
10. Kong EH, Evans LK, Guevara JP. Nonpharmacological intervention for agitation in dementia: a systematic review and meta-analysis. Aging Ment Health 2009;13(4): 512–20.
11. Seitz DP, Brisbin S, Herrmann N, et al. Efficacy and feasibility of nonpharmacological interventions for neuropsychiatric symptoms of dementia in long term care: a systematic review. J Am Med Dir Assoc 2012;13(6):503–6.e2.
12. Beck C, Ortigara A, Mercer S, et al. Enabling and empowering certified nursing assistants for quality dementia care. Int J Geriatr Psychiatry 1999;14:197–211.
13. Legg TJ, Adelman DS. Diagnosis: dementia. Psychiatric referral versus federal regulations: a balancing act for long-term care nurses. J Gerontol Nurs 2011; 37(11):24–7.
14. Center for Medicare and Medicaid Services. Federal regulations for long-term care facilities, title 42. 2012. Available at: http://www.cms.gov. Accessed May 1, 2012.
15. Food and Drug Administration. Black box warnings. 2012. Available at: http://www.fda.gov. Accessed May 1, 2012.
16. Stefanacci R. Evidence-based treatment of behavioral problems in patients with dementia. Ann Longterm Care 2008;16(4):33–5.
17. Lovheim H, Sandman PO, Karlsson S, et al. Sex differences in the prevalence of behavioral and psychological symptoms of dementia. Int Psychogeriatr 2009; 21(3):469–75.

18. Ballard CG, Corbett A, Chitramohan R, et al. Management of agitation and aggression associated with Alzheimer's disease: controversies and possible solutions. Curr Opin Psychiatry 2009;22:532–40.
19. Kaldy J. Solving the mystery by doing old-fashioned detective work. Provider 2012;38(7):25–37.
20. Kapusta P, Regier L, Bareham J, et al. Behaviour management in dementia. Can Fam Physician 2011;57:1420–2.
21. Koopmans RT, Zuidema SU, Leontjevas R, et al. Comprehensive assessment of depression and behavioral problems in long-term care. Int Psychogeriatr 2010; 22(7):1054–62.
22. Logsdon RG, McCurry SM, Teri L. Evidence-based psychological treatments for disruptive behaviors in individuals with dementia. Psychol Aging 2007;22(1): 28–36.
23. Lyketos CG, Carrillo MC, Ryan JM, et al. Neuropsychiatric symptoms in Alzheimer's disease. Alzheimers Dement 2011;7:532–9.
24. Williamson JE. Antipsyched out? McKnights. 2012. Available at: http://www.mcknights.com. Accessed May 1, 2012.
25. Cohen-Mansfield J. Agitated behavior in persons with dementia: the relationship between type of behavior, its frequency, and its disruptiveness. J Psychiatr Res 2008;43:64–9.
26. Zeller A, Hahn S, Needham I, et al. Aggressive behavior of nursing home residents toward caregivers: a systematic literature review. Geriatr Nurs 2009; 30(3):174–87.
27. Warchol K. Dementia care model facilitates quality outcomes. Aging Well 2012;5(2): 32. Available at: http://www.todaysgeriatricmedicine.com/archive/031912p32.shtml. Accessed November 8, 2013.
28. AGREE Trust (2012). Available at: http://www.agreetrust.org. Accessed March 1, 2012.
29. Liberati A, Altman DG, Tetzlaff J. The PRISMA statement for reporting systematic reviews and meta-analyses of studies that evaluate health care interventions: explanation and elaboration. Ann Intern Med 2009;151(4):W65–94.
30. Moher D, Hopewell S, Schulz KF. CONSORT 2010 explanation and elaboration: updated guidelines for reporting parallel group randomised trials. BMJ 2010; 340:c869.
31. Wiedenbach E. The helping art of clinical nursing. Current Nursing Web site. Available at: http://www.currentnursing.com/nursing_theory/Ernestine_Wiedenbach.html. Accessed March 1, 2012.
32. Hall GR, Buckwalter KC. Progressively lowered stress threshold: a conceptual model for care of adults with Alzheimer's disease. Arch Psychiatr Nurs 1987; 1(6):399–406.
33. James IA. Understanding behaviour in dementia that challenges: a guide to assessment and treatment. Philadelphia: Jessica Kingsley Publishers; 2011.
34. Boltz M, Capezuti E, Fulmer T, et al. Evidence-based geriatric nursing protocols for best practice. 4th edition. New York: Springer Publishing Company; 2012.
35. Fervers B, Burgers JS, Haugh MC, et al. Adaptation of clinical guidelines: literature review and proposition for a framework and procedure. Int J Qual Health Care 2006;18(3):167–76.

Index

Note: Page numbers of article titles are in **boldface** type.

A

Advanced practice registered nurse (APRN), proof-of-concept implementation of unit-based role, **1–13**
    components of team development, 8–10
    data collection, 10–11
    definition of, 4–5
    stages of team development, 10
    structural empowerment, 3–4
    team development components and solidification, 11–12
    team effectiveness, 5–8
    Vanderbilt Anticipatory Care Team, 2–3
Anticipatory care, with unit-based APRN role, 2–3
APRN. *See* Advanced practice registered nurse.

C

Cancer, colorectal, measuring endoscopic performance for quality improvement in prevention of, **15–27**
Catheter-associated urinary tract infection, diagnosis and treatment in adult neurocritical care patients, **29–43**
    appraisal of evidence and synthesis, 31–35
    background and significance, 29–30
    benefit to practice, 30–31
    conceptual framework, 31
    dissemination of project, 40
    future directions of project, 40
    practice setting, 30
    project results, 35–40
    purpose and specific aims, 30
Clinical competency, bridging gap between theory and, **69–80**
    combining the education strategies, 75–78
      for hospital staff development, 78
      in graduate education, 75–78
      in undergraduate education, 78
    concept mapping, 72–74
    meaningful learning, 71–72
    nurse-sensitive indicators, 70–71
    simulation, 75
Clinical practice guidelines, for behavioral problems in long-term care residents with dementia, **105–113**
    applicability to advanced practice, 111
    application of theory and framework, 109–110

Nurs Clin N Am 49 (2014) 115–121
http://dx.doi.org/10.1016/S0029-6465(13)00135-7
0029-6465/14/$ – see front matter © 2014 Elsevier Inc. All rights reserved.

nursing.theclinics.com

Moving?

Make sure your subscription moves with you!

To notify us of your new address, find your **Clinics Account Number** (located on your mailing label above your name), and contact customer service at:

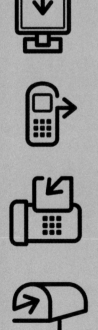

Email: journalscustomerservice-usa@elsevier.com

800-654-2452 (subscribers in the U.S. & Canada)
314-447-8871 (subscribers outside of the U.S. & Canada)

Fax number: 314-447-8029

Elsevier Health Sciences Division
Subscription Customer Service
3251 Riverport Lane
Maryland Heights, MO 63043

*To ensure uninterrupted delivery of your subscription, please notify us at least 4 weeks in advance of move.